# NUCLEAR CARDIOLOGY, THE BASICS

# CONTEMPORARY CARDIOLOGY

## CHRISTOPHER P. CANNON, MD
### SERIES EDITOR

# NUCLEAR CARDIOLOGY:
# THE BASICS

*How to Set Up and Maintain a Laboratory*

*by*

## FRANS J. TH. WACKERS, MD, PhD
*Yale University School of Medicine, New Haven, CT*

## WENDY BRUNI, BS, CNMT
*Yale–New Haven Hospital, New Haven, CT*

*and*

## BARRY L. ZARET, MD
*Yale University School of Medicine, New Haven, CT*

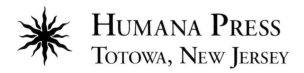

## HUMANA PRESS
### TOTOWA, NEW JERSEY

© 2004 Humana Press Inc.
999 Riverview Drive, Suite 208
Totowa, New Jersey 07512

**www.humanapress.com**

For additional copies, pricing for bulk purchases, and/or information about other Humana titles, contact Humana at the above address or at any of the following numbers: Tel.: 973-256-1699; Fax: 973-256-8341, E-mail: humana@humanapr.com; or visit our Website: http://humanapress.com

Due diligence has been taken by the publishers, editors, and authors of this book to assure the accuracy of the information published and to describe generally accepted practices. The contributors herein have carefully checked to ensure that the drug selections and dosages set forth in this text are accurate and in accord with the standards accepted at the time of publication. Notwithstanding, as new research, changes in government regulations, and knowledge from clinical experience relating to drug therapy and drug reactions constantly occurs, the reader is advised to check the product information provided by the manufacturer of each drug for any change in dosages or for additional warnings and contraindications. This is of utmost importance when the recommended drug herein is a new or infrequently used drug. It is the responsibility of the treating physician to determine dosages and treatment strategies for individual patients. Further it is the responsibility of the health care provider to ascertain the Food and Drug Administration status of each drug or device used in their clinical practice. The publisher, editors, and authors are not responsible for errors or omissions or for any consequences from the application of the information presented in this book and make no warranty, express or implied, with respect to the contents in this publication.

Cover illustrations provided by Dr. Frans J. Th. Wackers.

Cover design by Patricia F. Cleary.

This publication is printed on acid-free paper. ∞
ANSI Z39.48-1984 (American National Standards Institute) Permanence of Paper for Printed Library Materials.

Printed in the United States of America.   10   9   8   7   6   5   4   3   2   1

E-ISBN: 1-59259-426-3

Library of Congress Cataloging-in-Publication Data
Wackers, Frans J. Th.

>      Nuclear cardiology, the basics : how to set up and maintain a laboratory / by Frans J. Th. Wackers, Wendy Bruni, and Barry L. Zaret.
>              p.;cm.–(Contemporary cardiology)
>      Includes bibliographical references and index.
>      ISBN 0-89603-983-8 (alk. paper)
>      1. Heart–Radionuclide imaging. 2. Ambulatory medical care. 3. Medical laboratories. I. Bruni, Wendy. II. Zaret, Barry L. III. Title. IV. Contemporary cardiology (Totowa, N.J.:unnumbered)
>      [DNLM: 1. Heart–radionuclide imaging. 2. Laboratories–organization & administration. 3. Nuclear Medicine–standards. 4. Cardiovascular Diseases–radionuclide imaging. 5. Diagnostic Techniques, Cardiovascular–standards. 6. Radionuclide Imaging–standards. WG 23 W115n 2003]
>      RC683.5.R33W33 2003
>      616.1'207575–dc21                                                      2003049987

# PREFACE

In the United States the performance of nuclear cardiology studies continues to increase. As an example, in 1998, 4,160,739 myocardial perfusion imaging studies were done. In 2001 this number increased to 5,679,258. The nonhospital performance of perfusion imaging increased over the same time period from 1,188,731 to 1,789,207 studies (Arlington Medical Resources data). In 1999, there were approximately 1300 nonhospital sites with nuclear imaging capabilities, of which 600 were in physician's offices. By 2001, there were approximately 1700 nonhospital sites, of which 780 were in physician's offices (from IMV, LTD: http://www.imvlimited.com/mid/).

The growth of nuclear cardiology as an expanded outpatient laboratory enterprise is readily apparent. In the United States, as well as in other parts of the world, this growth has been linked to the recognition of the ability of cardiologists to perform these studies. The certification examination in nuclear cardiology is now well established in the United States. Accreditation of laboratories is also well established. Over the years, some of the most frequent questions asked by our former trainees relate to practical issues involved in the establishment of a nuclear cardiology laboratory. In view of the growth of the field, this is certainly not surprising.

There are a number of excellent texts on general nuclear cardiology available *(1–4)*. These books generally deal with the overall concepts of the field, its scientific basis, techniques, clinical applications, and clinical value. However, to our knowledge there does not presently exist a volume designed to provide the nuclear cardiologist with a manual dedicated to establishing and running a well-organized and state-of-the-art nuclear cardiology laboratory.

Consequently, the purpose of *Nuclear Cardiology: The Basics—How to Set Up and Maintain a Laboratory* is to provide the outline for the "nuts and bolts" establishment and day-today operation of a nuclear cardiology laboratory. In so doing, we have attempted to deal with the relevant issues that a laboratory director must address in either setting up the laboratory or in maintaining its competitive edge and clinical competence over time. We primarily attempt to identify issues related to outpatient imaging facilities. However, where appropriate, issues related to inpatients and hospital-based laboratories are also discussed.

*Nuclear Cardiology: The Basics—How to Set Up and Maintain a Laboratory* is aimed at cardiology fellows, nuclear cardiology fellows, and residents in nuclear medicine and radiology completing their training, as well as established cardiologists, radiologists, or nuclear physicians who want to establish a nuclear cardiology laboratory. The book should also be of value to nuclear cardiology technologists, laboratory managers, and health maintenance organizations. Attention has also been paid to those factors relevant for laboratory accreditation.

*Nuclear Cardiology: The Basics—How to Set Up and Maintain a Laboratory* is organized in what we feel is a logical progression. The initial chapter addresses what is required to establish the laboratory in terms of equipment, availability of radiopharmaceuticals, and staff qualifications. A chapter is devoted to the types of information patients should be provided with prior to arriving in the laboratory. Chapters are devoted to laboratory logistics and appropriate clinical protocols for stress studies. Several chapters deal with the technical aspects of performance of studies, such as those acquisition parameters relevant for high-quality studies, processing parameters, and quantification and display options. Examples are given of commonly encountered artifacts. We deal with issues relating to networking, both within one laboratory and linking several laboratories. Issues relating to dictation and reporting, coding and reimbursement, and quality assurance are also separately addressed. Finally, we address key policy issues that are relevant to high-quality clinical performance and conclude with a chapter addressing issues relevant to laboratory accreditation.

We are hopeful that *Nuclear Cardiology: The Basics—How to Set Up and Maintain a Laboratory* will fill an important clinical need within the cardiology and imaging communities. The book has been designed to be straightforward and to deal directly with the issues at hand. In many instances we present several sides of a particular issue. The final decision on which approach to take will depend on local circumstances.

In conclusion, it is very important to acknowledge the multiple lessons we have learned from the many technologists and trainees, in both cardiology and nuclear medicine, who have passed through our laboratory over the past two decades. Their input, as well as the opportunity to take part in their training, has helped us enormously in the conception and writing of this book.

***Frans J. Th. Wackers,*** MD, PhD
***Wendy Bruni,*** CNMT
***Barry L. Zaret,*** MD, PhD

### Selected Bibliography

1. Zaret BL, Beller GA (eds.) (1999). *Clinical Nuclear Cardiology, State of the Art and Future Directions.* Second Edition. Mosby, St. Louis, MO.

2. Iskandrian AE, Verani MS (eds.) (2003*). Nuclear Cardiac Imaging, Principles and Applications,* Third Edition, Oxford University Press, New York, NY.

3. Gerson MC (ed.) (1997). *Cardiac Nuclear Medicine,* Third Edition. McGraw-Hill, New York, NY.

4. Sandler MP, Coleman RE, Patton JA, Wackers FJTh, Gottschalk A (eds.) (2003). *Diagnostic Nuclear Medicine,* Fourth Edition. Lippincott Williams & Wilkins, Philadelphia, PA.

# CONTENTS

# ACKNOWLEDGMENTS

We are grateful for the invaluable work done by Donna Natale, CNMT, and Laurie Finta, RN, by providing help and expertise with the collection and formatting of the illustrations in this book. The help given by Mary Jo Zito, CNMT, and Vera Tsatkin, CNMT, is also much appreciated. We also acknowledge Barbara Williams, MD, Yi-Hwa Liu, PhD, and Patricia Aaronson for reviewing initial drafts of the manuscript and for providing valuable input. We also thank Ernest Garcia, PhD, Guido Germano, PhD, and Edward Ficaro, PhD, for providing us with illustrations of their proprietary software.

# Authors' Affiliations

## Frans J. Th. Wackers, MD, PhD

*Professor of Diagnostic Radiology and Medicine; Director, Cardiovascular Nuclear Imaging and Exercise Laboratories; Department of Diagnostic Imaging (Nuclear Cardiology); and Department of Medicine (Cardiovascular Medicine), Yale University School of Medicine, New Haven, CT*

## Wendy Bruni, CNMT

*Chief Technologist, Cardiovascular Nuclear Imaging and Exercise Laboratories, Yale–New Haven Hospital, New Haven, CT*

## Barry L. Zaret, MD, PhD

*Robert W. Berliner Professor of Medicine (Cardiovascular Medicine) and Professor of Diagnostic Radiology; Chief, Section of Cardiovascular Medicine; Associate Chair for Clinical Affairs, Department of Internal Medicine, Yale University School of Medicine, New Haven, CT*

# USING THIS BOOK AND THE COMPANION CD

All illustrations and movies in this book can be found in digital format on the accompanying CD. The images are best viewed on a high-resolution (1280 × 1280) color (24 bit or higher true color) computer monitor. The movies are best viewed at a display rate of 10 frames per second.

# 1 Getting Started

Whether planning a new nuclear cardiology imaging facility, or renovating an existing laboratory, there are many factors to be considered and many decisions to be made. This chapter will highlight and discuss many of these practical decisions.

The following issues will be considered:

- Physical space
- Equipment
- Radiopharmacy
- Additional miscellaneous supplies
- Staffing
- Radiation safety officer (RSO)

## PHYSICAL SPACE

The overall physical space and organization of a nuclear cardiology imaging facility must be such that patient confidentiality is protected in compliance with HIPAA regulations (see, www.hipaadvisory.com).

- **Imaging Rooms**
  Imaging rooms should be spacious enough to accommodate gamma camera systems. Currently a typical imaging room should be $14 \times 14$ ft at the minimum. (**Fig. 1-1.**) Cameras of different vendors differ in space requirements. It is important to know the footprint of the imaging system selected and that all equipment can be accommodated in the available space. "Hybrid" systems (e.g., SPECT-CT, PET-CT) require more space. If CT is used, lead shielding of the walls may be necessary.
- **Stress Rooms**—Stress rooms must be close to the imaging rooms. A typical stress room requires at a minimum $8 \times 8$ ft ($2.5 \times 2.5$ m). (**Fig. 1-2.**)

From: *Contemporary Cardiology: Nuclear Cardiology, The Basics*
F. J. Th. Wackers, W. Bruni, and B. L. Zaret © Humana Press Inc., Totowa, NJ

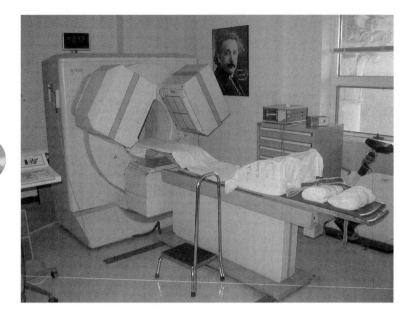

**Fig. 1-1.** Nuclear cardiology imaging room with triple-head gamma camera. After a patient is appropriately positioned on the imaging table, the table moves the patient feet-first into the gantry of the camera for SPECT image acquisition.

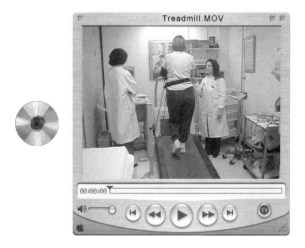

**Fig. 1-2.** Treadmill exercise testing. It is good medical practice to have two people present during an exercise test. One person, a physician or experienced nurse supervises the test and observes the ECG during exercise and operates the controls of the treadmill. Another person is present for taking and recording vital signs.

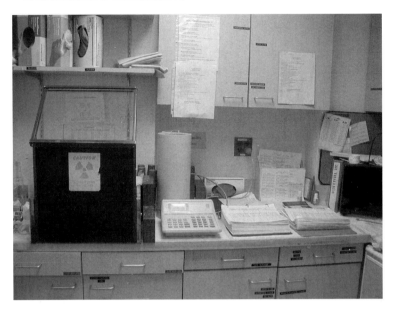

**Fig. 1-3.** Interior of the radiopharmacy, also known as hot lab. On the left is the lead-shielded work area. In the middle is the dose calibrator. On the right are the log books for recording the use of radioisotopes.

- **Injection Room**—The injection room is useful for the administration of radiopharmaceuticals when the patient is at rest. The minimum size required is 6 × 6 ft (1.8 × 1.8 m).
- **Patient Preparation Area**—This area is an option, but will facilitate the flow of patients, with 8 × 8 ft (2.5 × 2.5 m) being a minimum size.
- **Reception/Waiting Rooms and Toilet Facilities**—These areas should be sized so they are large enough for the expected patient volume.
- **Radiopharmacy**—This area is a necessity whether one plans for a fully operational "hot lab," or merely for the storage of "unit doses." Minimal required space is 6 × 6 ft (1.8 × 1.8 m). (**Fig 1-3**.)
- **Reading/Interpretation Area**—A separate and quiet area for interpretation of studies is optimal. In compliance with HIPAA regulations patient protected health information must be reviewed and discussed with consideration of patient confidentiality. This space also serves to preserve patient privacy and confidentiality.
- **Storage Area**—To store supplies, patient files, and digital image data.
- **Staff Area**—Areas for storage of personal items and for lunch breaks.
- **Office Space**—Offices for medical and technical directors.

# EQUIPMENT

## *Acquiring a Gamma Camera*

Before one begins to explore the options of different gamma cameras, one should decide on a number of important issues that may help focus the search.

- Will the camera be a *dedicated* cardiac gamma camera, or will general nuclear medicine imaging procedures be performed as well?
  *For dedicated cardiac cameras, one can purchase cameras with smaller field-of-view (FOV) heads.*
- How much physical space is available?
  *Does the gamma camera fit in the room? Is there enough work space around the camera?*
- Will only single-photon imaging or also coincidence or PET imaging be performed on the same gamma camera?
  *Not all equipment is capable of performing high-energy imaging. Thus, this may limit the choice of cameras. High-energy-imaging cameras are also more expensive.*

### HARDWARE CONSIDERATIONS

- **Size Field of View (FOV)**—If a camera will be used for other organ imaging in addition to cardiac imaging, a large FOV is needed. If the camera will be used only for nuclear cardiology imaging, a smaller FOV is appropriate.
- **Number of Heads**—Triple head or dual head gamma cameras are available. Dual heads are better for general nuclear medicine imaging; they are also cheaper.
- **Collimator Options**—Choose a collimator that will be adequate for the different acquisition needs anticipated.
- **PET/Coincidence Option**—This configuration requires thicker crystals, additional hardware/software, and reinforced gantry.
- **Attenuation Correction**—Additional hardware/software and radioactive sources are necessary for attenuation correction.
- **Automatic Collimator Change**—This feature is an excellent choice if collimators are to be changed frequently. However, close attention must be given to floor leveling.
- **Patient Table: Manual or Automatic**—The imaging table should be movable; this can be done by hand or with a motor. Some automatic tables have a motor mounted on the side of the table that juts out. This protruding part creates difficulties for stretcher patients and may affect the required room size. However, manual tables are difficult to move with obese patients and require exact floor leveling.

- **Table Limits**—Identify the maximal patient weight that the table can support. Consider the average weight of patients in the practice. Maximal acceptable patient weight is generally 350–400 lb (160–180 kg).
- **Gantry Size and Weight**—An engineer must authorize the floor's capacity to support the camera's weight. Reinforcement of the floor may be necessary, which adds to the overall cost of purchase and increases installation time.
- **Power Requirements**—Many gamma camera systems have special power needs. Check with the manufacturer.
- **Universal Power Supply (UPS)**—If outlet power fluctuates, one may need a UPS to maintain constant power for the gantry and to prevent system failures. Even if the power supply is stable, it is a good optional feature.
- **Computer Speed**—If quantitative processing is performed routinely, or if 16-bin ECG-gated studies are acquired, a fast(er) computer is required. The typical speed required is at least 2 GHz.
- **Computer Memory**—Most ECG-gated SPECT images are acquired with 8 frames per cardiac cycle. Extra memory is needed if 16-bin ECG-gated studies are acquired, or both stress and rest SPECT images are acquired in ECG-gated mode, or both. The typical amount of computer storage space and memory is > 4 GB.
- **Networking Capabilities**—Can the new system be networked to existing systems in the laboratory, and can image data be transferred back and forth? Does the system allow for remote and home reading? (See Chapter 16.)
- **Acquisition Terminal**—Is the acquisition terminal separate from the processing computer? Is there space in the room for the extra computer?
- **Service Issues**—Is there local service for the equipment? What is their average service response time? What is their backup or support? Talk to an area hospital or other area users that have the same service and ask about the average downtime of the camera, the service response times, and the service technician's capabilities. Negotiate for guaranteed minimal downtime.
- **Display Computer**—Cardiac SPECT imaging must be interpreted from a high-resolution (1280 × 1024 pixels) color monitor (24 bit or higher true color). Multiple color scales, including a linear gray scale, should be available. Cathode ray tube (CRT) monitors are superior. Flat panel monitors are at the present time still of lesser quality than CRTs.
- **Storage of Digital Data**—Computer memory and storage media are presently relatively cheap. Depending on volume of patient studies and ECG-gating parameters, one may need a large optical drive such as a 4.1 GB drive. Unprocessed and processed imaging data should be kept for

at least 3 yr or as regulated by state laws. When interpreting a study, it is considered good practice to compare the new study to previous ones.

## SOFTWARE CONSIDERATIONS

- **Quantitative Software**—Does the system provide adequate quantitative software programs? What are the choices? Are the programs validated in the literature? How much extra do they cost?
- **Display Options**—Are the display options easy to use and can they be modified to specific needs?
- **Ease of Learning**—Is the software user-friendly and easy to learn by the technical staff?
- **Applications**—Can a staff member go to classes to learn about the equipment and software? Does the vendor have application specialists that come on site to teach the technical staff how to use the equipment and software? If so, for how many days?
- **Quality Control (QC) Requirements**—How often is QC required and how easy can QC be performed?
- **Software Flexibility**—Is the software flexible? Can the software be manipulated easily to perform nonstandard tasks? Some software are written in a way that processing steps are strung together in "macros," which make it virtually impossible, or at least very difficult, to deviate from routine protocol. One should also consider whether software is in compliance with new HIPAA regulations. (See Chapter 16.)

## *Additional Ancillary Equipment*

### PRINTER

- **Networking Capabilities**—In a laboratory with multiple camera systems, it is important to purchase a printer that can be integrated into the local area network (LAN) and is capable of printing from all imaging equipment. Many imaging facilities routinely send hard copies of the images with the reports to referring physicians. Thus, a high-quality color laser printer is a good investment.
- **Quality**—Expensive glossy paper can be used to send hard copies to referring physicians and can also be used for teaching purposes and publications. For archiving and for documentation in the patient's chart, less expensive plain printing paper is also available.
- **Paper and Ink Cost**—Calculate the cost-per-print when comparing different systems.

### TREADMILL AND ECG MONITOR

- **Software Options**—Can the treadmill/ECG software easily be modified? Can laboratory-specific protocols be inserted in the program? Examples include printing ECGs at predetermined time intervals or the printing of certain parameters in the final report.

- **Test Setup**—Is the setup of a patient, i.e., entering patient information in computer, placement of electrodes, and arrangement of ECG cables, easily performed?
- **Bicycle Compatibility**—Can the ECG computer, if so required, operate in conjunction with bicycle exercise?
- **Cardiopulmonary Exercise Testing Compatibility**—With increasing numbers of patients with congestive heart failure, cardiopulmonary exercise testing with measurements of oxygen consumption has become a more common procedure *(1)*. Is the ECG computer compatible with cardiopulmonary testing equipment?
- **Stress Protocol Options**—Are all required exercise and pharmacological stress options available?
- **Treadmill Speed**—Does the treadmill start slowly enough so that the patient can step onto the belt easily?
- **Weight Limit**—Is the weight limit of the treadmill adequate for the majority of patients that will come for testing?

### INFUSION PUMP FOR PHARMACOLOGICAL STRESS

- **Ease of Use**—Make sure that the setup of the pump is easy and that infusion rates can be adjusted. This is especially important if dobutamine pharmacological stress is performed.
- **Infusion Rates**—The pump must have the ability to deliver over a wide range of infusion rates, so that patients of all body weights receive the appropriate doses. Smaller pumps may have preset infusion rates and are not adjustable. While these in general are very easy to use, they cannot be adequately adjusted for obese patients.
- **Syringe Compatibility**—Make sure the pump works with the brand of syringes used in the laboratory. Syringes of different brands have slightly different diameters. The pump must be adjustable to accommodate each particular brand of syringe.

### EXERCISE BICYCLE

- **Compatibility**—Is the bicycle compatible with the ECG computer equipment?
- **Ease of Use**—Can the bicycle seat be adjusted easily for patients of different heights? Is it easy to monitor and to change the Watts during stress?
- **Camera Compatibility**—If the bicycle is to be used in conjunction with exercise first-pass imaging, the handle bars must be removable so that the patient can be positioned close to the camera head.

### EMERGENCY EQUIPMENT

The following are required emergency equipment and drugs:

- Oxygen tank and regulator
- Nasal cannula and extension tubing
- Mouth piece
- Ambu bag
- Code cart and defibrillator
- Portable ECG monitor(s)
- Nitroglycerin tablets
- Aminophylline
- Lidocaine
- Atropine
- Metoprolol
- Aspirin
- Diltiazem
- Nebulizers
- Albuterol inhalers

The following are optional emergency drugs

- Furosemide
- IV Nitroglycerin
- Heparin

# RADIOPHARMACY

## *Setting up the Hot Lab*

Whether one decides to purchase technetium-99m generators and prepare radiopharmaceuticals on site in the laboratory, or to buy "unit doses" from a local commercial radiopharmacy, one needs to make sure that there is a separate and dedicated area for radiopharmaceutical preparation and storage, the "hot lab." The area is set aside from the usual work areas, has limited access, and therefore does not expose staff and patients to unnecessary radiation.

This area must be large enough to provide storage for both isotopes received and radioactive trash, and to allow for preparation and calibration of radiotracers (**Fig. 1-3**). The minimal size of a hot lab with a generator is approximately $6 \times 6$ ft ($1.8 \times 1.8$ m). For the handling of unit doses one needs to reserve an area of at least $4 \times 4$ ft ($1.2 \times 1.2$ m).

It is prudent to plan this component of the imaging facility with a radiation safety officer (RSO) and have him/her involved in the design of the facility from the very beginning. At least one cabinet, in which radioisotopes and radioactive trash are stored, requires walls with lead shielding. Whether or not the door and walls of the hot lab need lead shielding depends on what is being stored, where the hot lab is located, and the assessment of the RSO.

## SUPPLIES NEEDED FOR RADIOPHARMACY (WHETHER ONE USES A GENERATOR OR UNIT DOSES)

- **Radiation Caution Sign**—The door of the radiopharmacy, or area set aside as a radiopharmacy, must be marked with the standard radiation warning decal "Caution Radioactive Materials." (**Fig 1-4.**) Containers of radioactive material (lead pigs, syringes) must be marked with radiation warning labels. (**Fig. 1-5.**)
- **Dose Calibrator**—Some of the newer models come with "Radiopharmacy manager" computers. This program requires QC data to be entered prior to use on each working day. This eliminates forgotten QC. This ensures that QC is always up to date, which is crucial for the Nuclear Regulatory Commission (NRC) or a similar organizaton's inspections.
- **Cesium-137 Source**—Needed for daily QC of the dose calibrator (See Chapter 17.)
- **Lead Molybdenum Coddle**—Necessary for QC of technetium-99m from generators.
- **Dose Calibrator Dippers**—Multiple dippers should be available. A second or extra dipper is recommended in case the first dipper becomes contaminated.
- **Lead Shield with Glass**—Necessary for visual control when drawing up doses.
- **Lead bricks**—Used for additional shielding. Necessary for use with molybdenum-99 generators. (**Fig 1-6.**)
- **Lead Vials** Necessary if preparing radiopharmaceuticals.
- **Lead Pigs and Carrying Cases**—Necessary to reduce radiation exposure to personnel when carrying doses to different rooms.
- **Lead Syringe Shields**—Necessary to reduce technologist radiation exposure .
- **Lead-Lined Trash Containers**—Necessary to store radioactive trash. It is necessary to have a separate container for sharps/needles as well as one for all other waste.
- **Heat Block or Microwave**—Some radiopharmaceuticals kits, for example, sestamibi, require heating during preparation.
- **Refrigerator**—Some kits need to be refrigerated.
- **Long-Handled Tongs**—This is used to minimize radiation exposure when handling radiopharmaceutical kits.
- **Survey Meter**—This is mandatory for detecting spills and for performing daily room and trash surveys.
- **Syringes**—Various sizes may be needed depending on the type of radiopharmaceutical kits to be prepared.
- **Alcohol Pads**—These are necessary for drawing up doses, and for preparation of radiopharmaceutical kits under aseptic conditions.

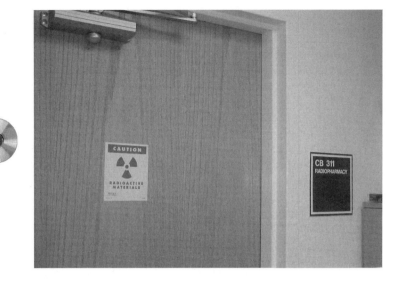

**Fig. 1-4.** Entrance door to radiopharmacy must be locked at all times and show caution sign for radioactive materials.

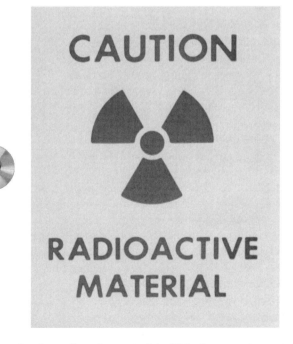

**Fig. 1-5.** Caution sign for radioactive materials. This sign must be posted at the entrance of all areas where radioactive materials are being used.

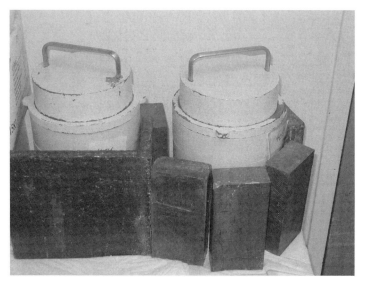

**Fig. 1-6.** Technetium generators and lead brick wall.

- **Gloves**—All radiopharmaceuticals must be handled with proper protective equipment.
- **Absorbent Pads**—These are useful to line counters and work area to absorb spills and make decontamination and spill containment easier.
- **Logbooks**—A logbook is needed for each isotope or radiotracer used. A logbook is also needed for dose calibrator QC, daily room surveys, molybdenum QC, package survey/receipt, wipe tests, and hot trash disposal (See Chapters 3 and 18.)
- **Labels**—All radiopharmaceutical vials and predrawn doses should be labeled.
- **Calculator**—This is necessary to calculate radiopharmaceutical decay, concentrations, and doses.

Additional supplies for radiopharmaceutical kit quality control are as follows:

- **Beakers**—To hold chemicals for chromatography.
- **Chemicals**  The type of chemical needed will vary depending on the radiopharmaceutical being prepared. Refer to the package insert for a list of chemicals needed.
- **Chromatography Paper**—Often used for QC of radiopharmaceutical kits. Refer to the package insert for specific instructions.
- **Ruler**—Used to mark chromatography paper for origin and cutting points.

## An Important Choice: Making Your Own Kits or Purchasing Unit Doses

For free-standing imaging facilities a practical arrangement to ensure a regular supply of radiopharmaceuticals may be through a contract with a regional commercial radiopharmacy. Radiopharmacies deliver precalibrated vials of quality-controlled radiopharmaceuticals, also known as "unit doses." The unit-dose approach is generally more expensive than the use of an on site generator.

It may be useful to compare the pros and cons of receiving unit doses versus preparing radiopharmaceuticals on site in an imaging facility. Cost and staffing are probably the two most important issues to consider. The price of molybdenum (Mo)-99 generators and of radiopharmaceutical kits depend on whether or not the imaging facility has a contract with a radiopharmaceutical vendor and also on the volume of patient studies. If the imaging facility has a contract with a radiopharmaceutical vendor, one may be entitled to discount pricing. In addition, the larger the patient volume, the better the price that can be negotiated. This is also true for unit dosing: the more doses one orders, the cheaper each dose will be. If price is a major factor, one should meet with local sales representatives and obtain quotes for the products.

Staff availability is also an important consideration. To elute the generator, to perform the QC, and to prepare the kits, a technologist has to come to the laboratory earlier in the morning than the rest of the technical staff. Depending on the number of kits to be made, this can take from 30 min to over 1 h. This technologist will be entitled to leave earlier at the end of the day than the rest of the staff . Therefore, one needs to have sufficient staff to be able to stagger shifts and to accommodate these hot lab duties.

Table 1-1 lists some other issues to be considered when deciding to order unit doses or to prepare radiopharmaceuticals on the premises.

## Preparing Radiopharmaceutical Kits on Site

If the decision is made to prepare radiopharmaceuticals on site in the imaging facility, written protocols must be in place that describe details of the procedures. For each specific brand of radiopharmaceutical separate protocols should exist. Kits from different vendors have different procedural steps and criteria. The protocol should meet the manufacturers' recommendations found in the package insert. The protocol should also detail radiation safety equipment and techniques to be used for the preparation of kits.

**Table 1-1**
**Considerations for Using Unit Doses or Making Kits**

| Consideration | Unit doses | Making kits |
|---|---|---|
| Staff time | Fast, no QC needed, except logging in delivery container. | Time consuming. |
| Lead brick shielding | Minimum needed: each dose comes individually shielded. | Need lead brick shields for both. |
| Lead waste containers | Few needed; syringes are usually returned to vendor. Small container may be needed for nonsharps waste. | Sharps and nonsharps containers will be needed as well as long-term storage space for longer lived radioisotopes. |
| Supplies | IV supplies needed. Some of the abovementioned hot lab supplies needed. | IV supplies, syringes, needles, and all abovementioned hot lab supplies needed. |
| Flexibility | Less flexible. Set delivery times. Sometimes an extra charge for doses ordered after scheduled delivery. | More flexible. Make kits and draw up doses as needed. |
| Changes | Doses are ordered the day before scheduled use. Sometimes a charge is applied for unused doses if there is patient cancellation. Doses cannot be adjusted for unexpected obese patients. | Changes in schedule and add-ons easily accommodateed. Doses can be adjusted when necessary. |
| Cost | Need large volume of patients to get cheapest price. Generally more expensive than making own kits. | Often cheaper than unit doses |

ADDITIONAL MISCELLANEOUS SUPPLIES

- **Caution Signs**—Doors of areas in which radioactive materials are stored or handled, or imaging is performed must be marked with the standard NRC radiation caution sign: "Caution Radioactive Material. (**Fig. 1-4.**)
- **Dosimeters**—Staff exposed to greater than 10% of occupational limits for radiation exposure must wear personal dosimeters, such as X-ray film badges, optically stimulated luminescent (OSL) or thermoluminescent dosimeters (TLD). These dosimeters should be read and changed on a monthly basis.
- **Table and Pillow Covering**—Compare cost of paper versus linen.
- **Gowns**—Necessary for patients who wear clothing with metal buttons.
- **Intravenous (IV) supplies**—Every patient who undergoes a stress test *must* have IV access and a running IV during the test. This is needed for the injection of the radiopharmaceutical at peak stress, and also for intravenous injection of pharmaceuticals in case of emergency. Patients who have rest imaging also need IV access for radiopharmaceutical administration.
- **ECG Leads**—Translucent chest leads are preferred for patients who will have subsequent imaging.
- **ECG Paper**—Sufficient amounts of ECG paper must be in stock.
- **Worksheets**—Worksheets are very useful for documentation by technologists and nurses of details and events during procedures. A separate worksheet may not be needed during treadmill exercise if the ECG computer generates a complete printable report. For pharmacological stress procedures, a chart is necessary on which one can record heart rate, blood pressure and ECG response, patient symptoms, and medication given. A worksheet that documents the radiotracer dose administered and time of administration, time imaging started, camera used, and other imaging parameters are important for QC. Additional notes by the technologist for the interpreting physician on patient height, weight, chest circumference, and bra size are also very useful. Sample stress worksheets are provided at the end of Chapter 5 and sample imaging worksheets can be found at the end of Chapter 6.
- **Charts**—Hard copy charts are still used for archiving purposes of recorded stress test parameters, ECGs, and images.

## LABORATORY STAFF

The staff of a nuclear cardiology imaging facility typically consists of a medical director, a technical director, medical staff, technical staff, radiation safety officer, stress testing personnel, and clerical staff. In smaller laboratories several functions may be fulfilled by one person.

## *Qualifications*

### NUCLEAR MEDICINE TECHNOLOGISTS

All nuclear medicine technologists should be either ARRT (N) (American Registry of Radiologic Technologists–Nuclear Medicine) or CNMT (Certified Nuclear Medicine Technologist) certified. At the present time there is a National Licensure Bill before the US Congress, which, if passed, will make it mandatory for all technologists to hold a current certification. For accreditation through the Intersocietal Commission for Accreditation of Nuclear Laboratories (ICANL), all nuclear medicine technologists should be licensed and obtain 15 h of VOICE credits (Verification of Involvement in Continuing Education) over 3 yr. Furthermore it is recommended that all technical staff be certified in cardiopulmonary resuscitation (CPR).

### ECG/STRESS TECHNOLOGISTS

Ideally stress technologists should be trained in exercise physiology. Unfortunately, these highly trained people are difficult to find. With additional on-site training in recording ECGs and administering stress tests, nuclear medicine technologists, emergency room technicians, or other medical technicians can be utilized as stress technologists. It is recommended that all technical staff be certified in basic life support (BLS).

### MONITORING STRESS TESTS

Physicians (cardiologists) usually monitor stress tests and interpret exercise ECGs. However personal physician supervision of all stress tests may be difficult to achieve in some laboratories. To facilitate the coverage of stress tests, physician-assistants and nurses with extensive cardiology experience, especially intensive care, can be trained to monitor stress tests and to interpret stress ECGs. Thus, whereas the type of personnel available in each laboratory may vary, it is important that adequate physician support is ensured in case of emergencies. A physician should always be near the stress testing area. For Medicare reimbursement for the performance of a stress test, "direct supervision" is required. That is, the physician must be in the immediate vicinity when the test is performed (see below). The staff supervising stress testing should be ACLS (Advanced Cardiac Life Support) certified.

In our laboratory stress testing routinely is administered by two persons (at least one with extensive training and experience in stress testing), one for operating the treadmill, watching the ECG, and communicating with the patient, and another person for recording vital signs (**Fig.1-2**).

MEDICAL STAFF INTERPRETING STUDIES

All nuclear cardiology studies should be interpreted by a qualified physician. The Intersocietal Commission for Accreditation of Nuclear Laboratories has defined the required training and credentials for nuclear cardiologists (see www.icanl.org). The medical director should have a current state medical license and be an Authorized User of radioisotopes. All interpreting medical staff should have current state medical licenses and preferably also be Authorized Users of radioisotopes. It is also recommended that all medical staff be certified in BLS or ACLS.

---

**Required Training and Experience for the Medical Director** (ICANL Standards)

The Medical Director must meet one or more of the following criteria:

A. Certification in nuclear cardiology by the Certification Board of Nuclear Cardiology (CBNC) (see www.cbnc.org), or
B. Board certified or Board eligible within 2 yr of finishing training in cardiology and completion of a minimum of a 4 mo formal training program in nuclear cardiology (Level 2 training according to the 2002 ACC/ASNC Revised COCATS Training Guidelines; see www.acc.org/clinical/training/cocats2.pdf). This is mandatory for cardiologists who began their cardiology training *in July 1995 or later*, or
C. Board certification in cardiology and training equivalent to Level 2 training, or at least 1 yr of nuclear cardiology practice experience with independent interpretation of at least 600 nuclear cardiology studies. This requirement applies only to cardiologists who began their cardiology training *before July 1995*, or
D. Board certified or Board eligible within 2 yr of finishing training in Nuclear Medicine, or
E. Board certified or Board eligible within 2 yr of finishing training in Radiology with at least 4 mo of nuclear cardiology training, or
F. Board certification in Radiology and at least 1 yr of nuclear cardiology practice experience with independent interpretation of at least 600 nuclear cardiology studies.
G. Ten years of nuclear cardiology practice experience with independent interpretation of at least 600 nuclear cardiology procedures.

Furthermore:

The Medical Director should obtain at least 15 h of AMA Category 1 CME credits relevant to nuclear cardiology every 3 yr. Yearly accumulated CME Credits should be kept on file and available for inspection.

The Medical Director is responsible for all clinical services provided and for the quality and appropriateness of care provided. The Medical Director may supervise the entire operation of the laboratory or delegate specific operations.

The interpreting medical staff are preferably CBNC-certified and have training and/or experience in nuclear cardiology as defined for the medical director. The interpreting medical staff should meet the same CME criteria as the medical director.

## *Physician Supervision of Diagnostic Tests*

Medicare regulation defines three levels of physician supervision: general, direct, or personal.

### GENERAL SUPERVISION

A procedure is performed under the physician's overall direction and control, but the physician's presence is not required during the performance of the procedure. The physician is responsible for protocols, policies and training of personnel who actually perform the test. Nuclear cardiology imaging procedures are performed under general supervision.

### DIRECT SUPERVISION

The physician must be present in the office and must be immediately available for assistance and direction throughout the performance of the procedure. It does not mean that the physician must be present in the room when the procedure is performed. Stress testing is performed under direct supervision.

### PERSONAL SUPERVISION

The physician must be present in the room during performance of the procedure.

## *Radiation Safety Officer (RSO)*

An imaging facility that uses radiopharmaceuticals must have a designated person who assumes the role of RSO and is responsible for the operation of the imaging facility within Federal or State regulations for radiation safety (see also Chapter 3).

The RSO can be either an authorized user according to NRC or state regulation (or individual country), or a qualified health physicist.

## *Authorized User*

The Nuclear Regulatory Commission (www.nrc.gov) has regulated the medical use of byproduct material. Authorized user means a physician who has fulfilled training requirements as outlined in NRC Regu-

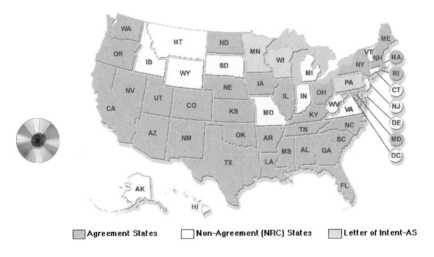

Agreement States          Non-Agreement (NRC) States          Letter of Intent-AS

Source: http://www.hsrd.ornl.gov/nrc/rulemaking.htm

**Fig. 1-7.** Map of 18 states that are under the regulatory authority of the Nuclear Regulatory Commission (non-agreement states), states that have entered an agreement with the NRC to discontinue regulatory authority by the NRC (agreement states), and states that have submitted letters of intent to become agreement states. (Source: http://www.Rsrd.ornl.gov/nrc/rulemaking.html)

lations 10 CFR part 35.290: Training for imaging and localization studies (or other country regulations).

## *How Does One Become an Authorized User?*

Since October 2002 new NRC training and experience requirements are in effect. In the 18 NRC, or nonagreement states (see **Fig. 1-7**), there are two pathways:

1. By completing a total of 700 h of classroom and laboratory training in specified subject areas and supervised work experience in areas specified in 10 CFR Part 35.290. See also ASNC web site (www.asnc.org) for details.
2. CBNC board certification.

Effective on October 24, 2002, the Nuclear Regulatory Commission recognizes CBNC certification in nuclear cardiology as evidence for adequate training (see also www.asnc.org for detailed description of training requirements).

In the 32 Agreement States, the following is required to become an authorized user: completion of 200 h of didactic training in radiation safety, 500 h of clinical experience, and 500 h of supervised work experience in radiation safety procedures. Agreement States have until October 24, 2005 to adopt regulations that are "essentially identical" (language from 10 CFR Part 35) to the training and experience requirements in 10 CFR Part 35.290.

The state of Florida requires Authorized User status to interpret nuclear medicine studies. In all other states Authorized User status has no connection with reading nuclear studies and reimbursement.

A list of NRC Agreement States can be found at www.hsrd.ornl.gov/nrc/rulemaking.htm.

## REFERENCE

1. Wasserman K, Hanson JE, Sue DY, Casaburi R, Whipp BJ (eds) (1999). Principles of exercise testing and interpretation. Third Edition, Lippincott Williams & Wilkins, Philadelphia, PA

# 2 Laboratory Logistics

The operation of a nuclear cardiology imaging facility requires planning, scheduling, and modifications that depend on the types of procedures and the number and type of patients referred for imaging.

In most imaging facilities two types of cardiac studies are performed:

- Radionuclide myocardial perfusion imaging
- Radionuclide angiocardiography

## MYOCARDIAL PERFUSION IMAGING

The majority of myocardial perfusion imaging procedures are performed in conjunction with either physical or pharmacological stress. The imaging procedure itself consists of two parts: post-stress imaging and rest or delayed imaging. Standard imaging protocols are described in detail in the Updated Imaging Guidelines for Nuclear Cardiology Procedures *(1)* (www.asnc.org menu: library and resources: guidelines and standards) We refer also to the Society of Nuclear Medicine Procedure Guidelines for Myocardial Perfusion Imaging (on line: www.snm.org).

The efficiency of a laboratory and its daily schedule are affected by the choice of stress procedures and imaging protocols. Tables 2-1 and 2-2 list typical stress and imaging procedures that may be performed in a cardiac imaging facility as well as the advantages and disadvantages of various imaging protocols. The availability of physicians or other medical staff to monitor stress test may also influence the choice of protocols.

### Time Requirements

The time requirements for both stress and imaging procedures are to be considered when making the daily laboratory schedule. Table 2-3 shows the time slots required for the various myocardial perfusion

From: *Contemporary Cardiology: Nuclear Cardiology, The Basics*
F. J. Th. Wackers, W. Bruni, and B. L. Zaret © Humana Press Inc., Totowa, NJ

**Table 2-1**
**Type of Stress Procedures**

*Physical Exercise*
Treadmill exercise
Bruce protocol
Modified Bruce protocol
Naughton protocol
Supine or upright bicycle exercise
Cardiopulmonary exercise testing
*Pharmacological Stress*
Dipyridamole vasodilation stress
Adenosine vasodilation stress
Dobutamine adrenergic stress

**Table 2-2**
**Type of Imaging Protocols**

*Thallium-201 (Tl-201) Perfusion Imaging*
One-day
Exercise–redistribution
Pharmacologic stress–redistribution
Rest (or reinjection)–redistribution
*Technetium-99m (Tc-99m) Agents (Sestamibi or Tetrofosmin) Perfusion Imaging*
Two-day
Rest only
Stress (exercise or pharmacologic) only
One-day (low dose-high dose)
Exercise–rest
Pharmacologic stress–rest
Rest–exercise
Rest–pharmacologic stress
*Dual Isotope Perfusion Imaging*
One-day
Rest Tl-201/stress Tc-99m Agent

imaging protocols, as well as the approximate total time required to perform each protocol.

From Table 2-3 it should be clear that the one-day imaging protocols with Tc-99m-labeled agents may be the most difficult protocols to fit into a daily schedule. However, if the stress study of a one-day protocol is unequivocally normal, a rest study is generally not needed (see below).

## *Logistical Advantages and Disadvantages of Various Myocardial Perfusion Imaging Protocols*

### Tl-201 one-day stress-redistribution

*Advantages*

> Widely used
> Cost is less than for Tc-99m-labeled agents
> High myocardial extraction fraction
> Good linearity of myocardial uptake versus blood flow

*Disadvantages*

> Relatively long half-life limits maximal dose to 4.5 mCi
> Substantial portion of photons in image are scattered photons
> Low-energy photons are easily attenuated and cause artifacts especially in obese patients and women with large breasts

### Tc-99m agent two-day stress-rest

*Advantages*

> Relatively high dose (20–30 mCi) administered; good count statistics and good quality
> Efficient protocol, if stress images are completely normal, and clinical and exercise parameters do not suggest coronary artery disease, no rest study may be needed
> Good quality ECG-gated study due to high dose

*Disadvantages*

> Takes two days to get final results
> Inconvenient, patient needs to come to the laboratory on two separate days

### Tc-99m agent one-day stress first-rest second

*Advantages*

> All stress testing is done in the morning. This may be more convenient depending on physician practice patterns (e.g., physicians seeing patients in the afternoon)
> Efficient protocol: if stress images are completely normal, and clinical and exercise parameters do not suggest coronary artery disease, no rest study may be needed

*Disadvantages*

> Relatively low-count-density stress images
> (first injection is low dose)
> Low-count-density ECG-gated stress images
> Not feasible in obese patients
> Long time required to complete entire stress–rest study (5–6 h)

### Tc-99m agent one-day rest first-stress second

*Advantages*

> High-count-density stress images (second injection is high dose)
> Good-quality ECG-gated images

**Table 2-3**
**Myocardial Perfusion Imaging**[a]

*One-Day Tl-201 Protocols*

| | | | | | | | | Total Time (min) |
|---|---|---|---|---|---|---|---|---|
| Tl-201 Ex-Red | Ex 30 min | Ex inj/Int 10 min | Ex SPECT 30 min | Red Int 180 min | Red SPECT 30 min | | | 280 |
| Tl-201 PhSt-Red | PhSt 45 min | PhSt inj/Int 10 min | PhSt SPECT 30 min | Red Int 180 min | Red SPECT 30 min | | | 295 |
| Tl-201 Rest-Redist | R inj 10 min | R inj/Int 10 min | R SPECT 30 min | Red Int 240 min | Red SPECT 30 min | | | 320 |

*One-Day Tc-99m Protocols*

| | | | | | | | | Total Time (min) |
|---|---|---|---|---|---|---|---|---|
| Tc-99m 1day Ex-R | Ex 30 min | Ex inj/Int 15 min | Ex SPECT 30 min | Int 120 min | R inj R 10 min | inj/Int 45 min | R SPECT 30 min | 280 |
| Tc-99m 1day R-Ex | R inj 10 min | R inj/Int 45 min | R SPECT 30 min | Int 120 min | Ex 30 min | Ex inj/Int 15 min | Ex SPECT 30 min | 280 |
| Tc-99m 1day PhSt-R | PhSt 45 min | PhSt inj/Int 45 min | PhSt SPECT 30 min | Int 120 min | R inj 10 min | R inj/Int 45 min | R SPECT 30 min | 325 |
| Tc-99m 1day R-PhSt | R inj 10 min | R inj/Int 45 min | R SPECT 30 min | Int 120 min | PhSt 45 min | PhSt inj/Int 45 min | PhSt SPECT 30 min | 325 |

*continued*

## Table 2-3 (*Continued*)
## Myocardial Perfusion Imaging[a]

### Two-Day Tc-99m Protocols

| | | | | | | Total Time (min) |
|---|---|---|---|---|---|---|
| Tc-99m Ex* | Ex 30 min | Ex inj /Int 15 min | Ex SPECT 30 min | | | 75 |
| Tc-99m PhSt* | PhSt 45 min | PhSt inj/Int 45 min | PhSt SPECT 30 min | | | 120 |
| Tc-99m R* | R inj 10 min | R inj/Int 45 min | R SPECT 30 min | | | 85 |

### Dual Isotope Rest Tl-201/Stress Tc-99m Agent Protocols

| | | | | | | | | Total Time (min) |
|---|---|---|---|---|---|---|---|---|
| Dual Isot 1day R-Ex | R inj 10 min | R inj /Int 30 min | R SPECT 30 min | Int 10 min | Ex 30 min | Ex inj /Int 15 min | Ex SPECT 30 min | 155 |
| Dual Isot 1day R-PhSt | R inj 10 min | R inj /Int 30 min | R SPECT 30 min | Int 10 min | PhSt 45 min | PhSt inj /Int 45 min | PhSt SPECT 30 min | 200 |

[a]Abbreviations: Ex=exercise; PhSt=pharmacological stress; R=rest; Red=redistribution; inj=injection; Int=interval; min=minutes; Isot=isotope; *=Ex performed on one day and R performed on a different day.

All stress testing is done in the afternoon. This may be more convenient depending on physician practice patterns (e.g., physicians seeing patients in the morning)

*Disadvantages*

Stress coverage needed in the afternoon

Long time required to complete rest–stress study (5–6 h)

**Dual isotope Tl-201rest/Tc-99m stress**

*Advantages*

Fast protocol, < 3 h for complete study

High count stress study

Good quality ECG-gated stress study

*Disadvantages*

Comparison of myocardial distribution of two different isotopes with different physical characteristics which may affect image pattern

## *Daily Schedule for Stress Testing and Imaging*

The time slots that are shown in Table 2-3 should be considered when making a daily work schedule. Creating an efficient patient schedule can be a substantial challenge, particularly because defined time intervals are required between the two myocardial perfusion imaging sessions.

The schedule for cardiac nuclear imaging is unique in that it does not consist of just a series of consecutive patient exams; each patient often requires two imaging sessions (stress and rest), separated by a time interval of a number of hours. In order to use the time intervals between the two imaging sessions efficiently, patient examination should be staggered.

The following examples are provided for an imaging facility with one exercise treadmill and one gamma camera. Depending on patient volume, for increased efficiency it may be better to have one technologist perform imaging, and another person (e.g., exercise physiologist, technologist, or physician) perform the injections of radiopharmaceuticals (during stress and at rest). With increasing numbers of treadmills and gamma cameras, the schedules are more complicated. In addition, a schedule depends on the type of stress and imaging protocols performed.

The simplest patient imaging schedule is a two-day schedule for a one gamma camera imaging facility.

The schedules below are for a laboratory that uses a Tc-99m-labeled radiopharmaceutical for both rest and stress imaging and a two-day schedule.

It should be noted that in these examples it is assumed that the patient arrives at the appointment time and that it takes 30 min to prepare and stress the patient. The patient is injected 30 min after arrival and imaged 30 min after injection. The rest images are acquired 45 min after injection of the radiopharmaceutical. Patients A,B,C, and D are patients who have their stress tests and stress imaging on this day. Patients 1,2,3, and 4 had a stress test the previous day and return on this day for rest imaging.

---

**Example of two-day imaging schedule**

| | | | |
|---|---|---|---|
| 8:00 AM | Stress pt. A | 9:00 AM | Image pt. A |
| 8:45 AM | Stress pt. B | 9:45 AM | Image pt. B |
| 9:30 AM | Stress pt. C | 10:30 AM | Image pt. C |
| 10:15 AM | Stress pt. D | 11:15 AM | Image pt. D |
| 11:00 AM | Stress pt. E | 12:00 PM | Image pt. E |

*Lunch*

| | | | |
|---|---|---|---|
| 12:30 PM | Inject Rest pt. 1 | 1:15 PM | Image pt.1 |
| 1:00 PM | Inject Rest pt. 2 | 1:45 PM | Image pt.2 |
| 1:30 PM | Inject Rest pt. 3 | 2:15 PM | Image pt.3 |
| 2:00 PM | Inject Rest pt. 4 | 2:45 PM | Image pt.4 |
| 2:30 PM | Inject Rest pt. 5 | 3:15 PM | Image pt.5 |

---

The following is an example of the schedule for the same laboratory for a 1-day imaging schedule. The same assumptions as shown above for the two-day schedule, i.e., times required for patient preparation, and time intervals after injections and for imaging are taken into account. Patients 1,2,3,4, and 5 all have a same day imaging protocol. Patients 1 and 2 have rest imaging first, whereas patients 3,4, and 5 have the stress portion first.

---

**Example of one-day imaging schedule**

| | | | |
|---|---|---|---|
| 7:30 AM | Inject Rest pt. 1 | 8:15 AM | Image (rest) pt.1 |
| 8:00 AM | Inject Rest pt. 2 | 8:45 AM | Image (rest) pt. 2 |
| 8:15 AM | Stress pt. 3 | 9:15 AM | Image (stress) pt. 3 |
| 9:00 AM | Stress pt. 4 | 10:00 AM | Image (stress) pt. 4 |
| 9:45 AM | Stress pt. 5 | 10:45 AM | Image (stress) pt. 5 |
| 10:30 AM | Stress pt. 1 | 11:30 AM | Image (stress) pt. 1 |
| 11:15 AM | Stress pt. 2 | 12:15 PM | Image (stress) pt. 2 |

*Lunch*

| | | | |
|---|---|---|---|
| 12:45 PM | Inject Rest pt. 3 | 1:30 pm | Image (rest) pt. 3 |
| 1:30 PM | Inject Rest pt. 4 | 2:15 PM | Image (rest) pt. 4 |
| 2:15 PM | Inject Rest pt. 5 | 3:00 PM | Image (rest) pt. 5 |

The details of a daily schedule of procedures and tests differ from laboratory to laboratory, owing to the radiopharmaceuticals and protocols used, and to the availability of physicians to monitor stress tests.

For example, if physicians have office hours in the morning, it may be practical and convenient to perform rest imaging, as shown below, in the morning and stress testing in the afternoon.

---

### Example of one-day imaging schedule (rest studies first in the morning)

| | | | |
|---|---|---|---|
| 8:00 AM | Inject Rest pt. 1 | 8:45 AM | Image (rest) pt.1 |
| 8:30 AM | Inject Rest pt. 2 | 9:15 AM | Image (rest) pt.2 |
| 9:00 AM | Inject Rest pt. 3 | 9:45 AM | Image (rest) pt.3 |
| 9:30 AM | Inject Rest pt. 4 | 10:15 AM | Image (rest) pt.4 |
| 10:00 AM | Inject Rest pt. 5 | 10:45 AM | Image (rest) pt.5 |
| 10:30 AM | Inject Rest pt. 6 | 11:15 AM | Image (rest) pt.6 |
| *Lunch* | | | |
| 11:15 PM | Stress pt. 1 | 12:15 PM | Image (stress) pt.1 |
| 12:00 PM | Stress pt. 2 | 1:00 PM | Image (stress) pt.2 |
| 12:45 PM | Stress pt. 3 | 1:45 PM | Image (stress) pt.3 |
| 1:30 PM | Stress pt. 4 | 2:30 PM | Image (stress) pt.4 |
| 2:15 PM | Stress pt. 5 | 3:15 PM | Image (stress) pt.5 |
| 3:00 PM | Stress pt. 6 | 4:00 PM | Image (stress) pt.6 |

---

## EQUILIBRIUM RADIONUCLIDE ANGIOCARDIOGRAPHY (ERNA)

Although radionuclide myocardial perfusion imaging is the most frequently performed imaging modality, in many laboratories equilibrium radionuclide angiocardiographies (ERNAs) are performed to assess left ventricular function in a variety of clinical circumstances. In our laboratory ERNAs are frequently requested for 1) oncology patients before and during the course of therapy with potentially cardiotoxic drugs, 2) for evaluation of patients with cardiomyopathy or recent infarction, and 3) to follow the effect of therapy in patients with abnormal left ventricular function.

### *Time Requirements*

Tables 2-4 and 2-5 show the time slots required for rest and rest–exercise ERNA protocols, as well as the approximate total time required to perform the protocols. It is assumed that in vitro kits are used for labeling of the patient's red blood cells. (Refer to Chapters 8 and 9 for complete discussion of ERNA imaging procedures.)

## Table 2-4
## Rest Equilibrium Radionuclide Angiocardiography

| Rest ERNA | iv line | Draw blood | Label blood | Reinject blood | Imaging | Total time |
|-----------|---------|------------|-------------|----------------|---------|------------|
| Planar | 10 min | 1 min | 20 min | 1 min | 30 min | 62 min |
| SPECT | 10 min | 1 min | 20 min | 1 min | 40 min | 72 min |

## Table 2-5
## Rest–Exercise Equilibrium Radionuclide Angiography[a]

| R-Ex ERNA | Blood labeling | Rest ERNA | Stress Set-up | Ex ERNA Stage1 | Ex ERNA Stage 2 | Ex ERNA Stage "n" | Post Ex ERNA | Total time |
|-----------|----------------|-----------|---------------|----------------|-----------------|-------------------|--------------|------------|
| Planar | 30 min | 30 min | 30 min | 3 min | 3min | 3xn min | 3 min | 102+ min |

[a]Note: Rest–exercise ERNA is shown for completeness. In actual practice exercise ERNAs are currently infrequently performed in most laboratories.

### FITTING ERNAS INTO THE DAILY SCHEDULE

Fitting ERNAs into the daily laboratory schedule is usually relatively easy if the ERNA volume is small. If the gamma camera used for myocardial perfusion imaging is also used for ERNAs, the most practical approach is to schedule ERNAs either at the beginning or at the end of the working day.

It is generally not practical to attempt to "squeeze" ERNAs between two myocardial perfusion studies in the course of the day. A complex schedule has the unavoidable tendency to run behind in time. A schedule that is too tight also causes problems and undesirable delays.

Obviously if the laboratory has a dedicated gamma camera for ERNAs, there is no interference with the general daily schedule.

### REFERENCE

1. DePuey GE, Garcia EV (eds) (2001). Updated imaging guidelines for nuclear cardiology procedures, Part I. *J Nucl Cardiol* 8;G1–58.

# 3    Radiation Safety

Radiation safety is an extremely important issue for nuclear cardiology laboratories. It is mandatory that imaging facilities operate in compliance with Nuclear Regulatory Commission regulations (www.nrc.gov) and/or those imposed by the state and local agencies in states not directly under NRC supervision ("agreement states") or similar agencies in other countries.

## RADIATION SAFETY OFFICER

It is the responsibility of a radiation safety officer (RSO) to ensure that the daily operation of a nuclear cardiology imaging facility is in compliance with radiation safety regulations. A RSO should help in developing policies and procedure protocols for radiation safety. The RSO should provide input with the set-up of the hot lab area and should ensure that all necessary areas are adequately lead-shielded. Furthermore, the RSO will make sure that all necessary equipment for handling and monitoring of radioactive materials is available. The RSO will also help in monitoring the radiation exposure of patients, staff, and environment such that exposure levels are as low as reasonably achievable (ALARA). The RSO also may help in setting up guidelines for patient dosing. Written protocols and policies should be in place to ensure compliance with regulations. Responsibilities of a RSO are listed in Table 3-1.

From: *Contemporary Cardiology: Nuclear Cardiology, The Basics*
F. J. Th. Wackers, W. Bruni, and B. L. Zaret © Humana Press Inc., Totowa, NJ

**Table 3-1**
**The Role of a RSO Generally Consists of the Following**

Instruction and training of personnel in radiation safety
Monitoring personnel radiation exposure
Radiation safety of facility and equipment
Incident response (overexposure, spills, etc.)
Security of licensed material
Radiation surveys
Radioactive material inventory records
Radioactive waste management
Maintenance of appropriate records and reports concerning radiation safety

---

**How to find a RSO for a new imaging facility?**

A RSO can be either a physician who is an authorized user according to the appropriate governing regulations, or a health physicist with special training as a RSO.

RSOs are often willing to serve as part-time consultants to free-standing imaging facilities.

Information may be available by contacting:
- Local hospitals with a RSO
- State Health Agencies
- American Association of Physicists in Medicine (www.aapm.org)
- Health Physics Society (www.hps.org)

---

A list of the recommended policies with regard to radiation safety that should be in place in a nuclear cardiology imaging facility *(1)* is given in Table 3-2. These are also required for ICANL accreditation (see Chapter 21).

## *Molybdenum-99 Check*

After eluting a generator, the Tc-99m eluant must be checked for contamination with Mo-99. The limit of μCi of Mo-99 per mCi of Tc-99m is set by the RSO. If the limit is exceeded, the Tc-99m eluant should not be used. The NRC-recommended limit for Mo-99 contamination is 1 μCi of Mo-99 per mCi of Tc-99m, not to exceed 5 μCi Mo-99 per dose.

## *Dose Calibrator Daily Constancy Check*

This quality assurance should be done daily prior to using the dose calibrator. Normally, a Cs-137 source is measured in the dose calibrator and the amount of activity is recorded. This measurement will alert the

## Table 3-2
## Recommended Policies for Radiation Safety

Molybdenum-99 check (only in laboratories that elute technetium-99m generators)
Dose calibrator daily constancy check
Radioactive package receipt
Daily survey of trash and work areas
Weekly wipe test of all work areas
Radioactive spill containment and decontamination
Disposal and storage of radioactive hot trash
Accuracy and linearity testing of dose calibrator
Calibration of survey meter

user if there is a calibration problem. The RSO can set the limits for acceptable measurements.

## *Radioactive Package Receipt*

All radioactive packages must be surveyed and undergo wipe tests prior to opening to ensure that the package is not contaminated. It is also a good idea to do a wipe test of the lead container inside the package to make sure that it is not contaminated. A written policy describing a protocol for receiving and handling of radioisotopes should be present. The written policy should state what to do in the event the package is contaminated.

## *Daily Survey of Trash and Work Areas*

At the end of each day all trash, linen carts, and work areas should be surveyed to detect any radioactive spills that may have occurred. Any work surfaces found to be contaminated should be cleaned according to the radioactive spill policy and then resurveyed. If the area is still contaminated, it may need to be sealed off and resurveyed in the morning prior to use. Any trash or linen found to be contaminated should be held for decay following local hot trash policy. A log of the daily surveys should be kept on hand.

## *Weekly Wipe Test of all Work Areas*

Each week all work areas (i.e., counters and adjacent floor where radiotracers are placed or used, treadmills, and so forth) where contamination is possible should be wipe tested. Any areas found to be contaminated should be cleaned in accordance with the radioactive spill policy and then rewiped. If the area is still contaminated, it may need to be sealed off and rewiped in the morning prior to use.

## Radioactive Spill Containment and Decontamination

This written policy should describe how to contain and decontaminate a radioactive spill using the proper radiation safety equipment. It should also specify the limits that indicate the area is usable or that the area needs to be sealed off until contamination has decayed to the proper level. The policy should also list who to contact in the event of a radioactive spill.

## Disposal and Storage of Radioactive Hot Trash

All radioactive trash must be held for decay before it can be discarded. The policy should discuss where the trash is stored, how it is to be labeled, the acceptable level at which it can be discarded safely, and where to discard it.

## Accuracy and Linearity Testing of Dose Calibrator

Depending on local regulations or on the RSO's requirements, this testing is done either quarterly or yearly. This quality control test helps to ensure that the dose calibrator is working properly.

## Calibration of Survey Meter

This test is usually done by the RSO or can be done by an independent company annually. It is important to determine that the survey meter is functioning properly.

## Personnel Dosimeter

Individuals who receive more than 10% of the quarterly limits of radiation exposure for occupational workers must wear dosimeters. These may consist of X-ray film badges, optically stimulated luminescence (OLS) dosimeters, or thermoluminescent dosimeter (TLD) rings.

Technical staff who become pregnant must declare their pregnancy in writing to the employer. The radiation exposure of pregnant personnel must be monitored and is limited to 50 mrem/mo during the pregnancy. No other special protection is required. To meet this limit, it may be necessary to have the pregnant mother refrain from hot lab duties and injections, since this is when the technologists obtain most of their exposure. Being pregnant does not impede a technologist's ability to perform imaging of patients.

## REFERENCE

1. Bushberg JT, Leidholdt EM. Radiation Protection,Chapter 9, in: Sandler MP, Coleman RE, Patton JA, Wackers FJTh, Gottschalk A (eds.) (2003) Diagnostic Nuclear Medicine, Fourth Edition, Lippincott Williams & Wilkins, Philadelphia, PA.

# 4 Patient Preparation

Patients should be well informed about what to expect during the nuclear cardiology procedure. In order to decrease the number of rescheduled and canceled appointments, it is important to make sure patients are not only properly prepared for the procedure, but also that they are well informed about the examination. They should be informed about all aspects, including the duration of the procedure, *before* they arrive in the laboratory.

This chapter discusses:

- Patient preparation
- Preparation for stress protocols

The following is the minimum information that should be communicated to a patient:

1. Date and time of test.
2. Directions and parking information.
3. Location of imaging facility.
   *Preparation for procedure*:
4. Light meal or fasting on morning of test.
5. Possible discontinuation of medication in consultation with referring physician.
6. Notify patients not to drink coffee or caffeine-containing beverages on morning of test (Table 4-1).
7. Wear comfortable clothing and rubber-soled shoes or sneakers.
   *Very important*:
8. Information about total duration of stress and imaging test.
9. Notify male patients that some chest hair may be shaved for ECG electrode placement.
10. Advise that IV line will be inserted in forearm.
11. Explain purpose and end point(s) of stress test.

From: *Contemporary Cardiology: Nuclear Cardiology, The Basics*
F. J. Th. Wackers, W. Bruni, and B. L. Zaret © Humana Press Inc., Totowa, NJ

12. Provide information when the referring physician can be expected to have the results of the test. *Emphasize that results will be reported quickly to the physician.*

Additional relevant information for patients can be found on the ASNC website: The first is titled "An Overview of Nuclear Cardiology" located at http://www.asnc.org/aboutnc/overview.htm on the ASNC website; and the second is titled "Nuclear Cardiology Patient Information" and can be found at http://www.asnc.org/aboutnc/brochure.htm. Both documents can be printed and made available to patients.

## PATIENT PREPARATION

The preparation of patients for stress procedures is different depending on the stress modality, i.e., physical exercise or pharmacological stress. For both stresses it is recommended that the patient is fasting and has an empty stomach. For pharmacological stress the patient must abstain from caffeine-containing beverages or food on the day of the procedure.

---

There is a practical advantage to giving **identical preparatory instructions** to every patient regardless of whether they are scheduled for physical exercise or for pharmacological stress. Frequently, a patient's ability to exercise is overestimated and an adequate exercise end point cannot be reached. A patient scheduled for an exercise test can be switched readily to pharmacological stress if he/she received the same instructions as a patient scheduled for pharmacological stress.

---

## DISCONTINUATION OF MEDICATION

Depending on the indication for stress testing and the clinical question to be answered, it may be advisable to discontinue medication such as beta-blockers, calcium-blockers medication and long- and short-acting nitrates before the procedure. For example, if a patient is referred for the *diagnosis* of coronary artery disease, medication probably can be stopped. However, if a patient has known coronary artery disease, the purpose of the test may be to evaluate the patient on his/her daily medical regimen. *The decision to temporarily stop medication should always been done in consultation with the referring physician.*

If the test is performed for diagnostic purposes, beta-blocking and calcium-blocking medications preferably should be stopped 24 h before, or at the least on, the day of the procedure. Nitrates should not be taken on the day of the procedure.

Diabetic patients should take their regular dose of insulin and a light breakfast on the morning of the procedure.

## BREAST FEEDING MOTHERS

At times it may be medically indicated to perform radionuclide imaging in breast feeding mothers. Radioisotopes are excreted in breast milk and expose the infant to radiation. The radiation safety approach is to either pump the breasts before the injection of radioisotope and store the milk, or if this is not feasible, collect milk and allow for appropriate decay before giving the milk to the infant. Breast milk can be stored in the refrigerator for 5 d, or frozen for up to 6 mo. The physician or RSO should determine how long (e.g., 48 h for Tc-99m-agents) the milk should be stored for adequate decay. There is no need to discard the milk. For exams that are scheduled ahead of time, the policy and method should be explained to nursing mother. It is not always possible to pump ahead of time. Consequently, it is important to discuss the storage and time required for decay with the mother prior to performing the imaging procedure.

---

**Example of patient appointment information sheet that can be mailed to a patient before the procedure.**

APPOINTMENT(S):

    DATE: _____ TIME: _____

    DATE: _____ TIME: _____

    Please arrive 15 minutes prior to your scheduled appointment for registration and                         insurance purposes.

PLACE:

- (address of imaging facility)
- Take the "C" elevators to the xth floor, room XXXX (directly across from the elevator).

    Park in the parking garage and bring your parking ticket with you to be validated.

HOW LONG WILL IT TAKE?

    The test consists of two parts: Each portion takes approx 2 h with a 1 1/2– 3 h break between the two parts depending on the exam scheduled.

PREPARATION:

- ABSOLUTELY NO caffeine or decaffeinated beverages 12 h before the test (including coffees, teas, sodas, and chocolates). You may eat a light breakfast (small bowl of cereal OR toast and juice) up to 2 h before your test.

---

- If you have diabetes, eat normally (remember NO caffeine or decaf) and take your insulin.
- Wear comfortable clothing and rubber sole shoes

PRECAUTIONS:

If you think you may be pregnant or if you are breast feeding, please tell your doctor immediately.

MEDICATIONS:

Unless instructed by your doctor, continue to take your medication(s).

If you are taking theophylline or any other asthma or emphysema medication, please contact your doctor as it MAY need to be discontinued 48 h before the test.

WHAT CAN YOU EXPECT:

- The two parts of the test consist of a STRESS study and a REST study. The stress OR the rest study can be done first and will depend on the type of exam you have been scheduled for.
- The stress test will require that ECG leads be placed on your chest to monitor your heart rate. A small dose of a radioactive tracer will be injected through an IV in your arm and images of your heart will be taken for approx 45 min.

  There are no side effects to the injection. However, if you think you are pregnant, please inform the technologist immediately.
- The rest study will consist of another injection of the radioactive tracer through the IV and a second set of images to be taken of your heart.
- There will be a break between the stress and rest portions of the test. The break ranges from 1 1/2 to 3 h depending on the type of study you are having. The technologist will tell you when you need to return and what restrictions, if any, there are for eating.
- The test may be completed in one day OR over two days. If you are scheduled to have the test over two days, the stress is done on one day and the rest is done on the other. It does not matter which is done first.

  Please refer to the appointment section to see when you are scheduled to have your test.

HOW DO YOU GET TEST RESULTS?

A nuclear cardiologist will study all the images and ECGs, prepare a report, and send it to your physician. This may take one or two days. Your personal physician will discuss the results with you and what they mean for your health. If your study is abnormal, the cardiologist may call your physician immediately.

If you have any concerns or questions about your appointment, you can call the Cardiology Stress Laboratory at 999-999-9999.

# CONSENT FOR STRESS TESTING

Although the risk for adverse effects due to stress testing is low, it is not nonexistent. In many facilities the patient is asked to sign a consent form prior to the procedure. A sample consent form for stress testing is shown in the accompanying box.

---

**Cardiovascular Nuclear Imaging
and Exercise Laboratory**

99 Main St., City, CT 9999            ph: (999) 999-9999

Consent for Stress Testing

I am scheduled to undergo a cardiac stress test.

I understand that this test involves walking or running on a treadmill.

I understand that this test involves the infusion of a medication that stresses the heart.

During the test I will be watched for symptoms and monitored by an electrocardiogram. In addition heart rate and blood pressure measurements will be taken.

I understand that certain complications may occur including, but not limited to, heart attack, heart rhythm abnormality, stroke and death. I also understand that physical trauma may be incurred during the performance of the test.

The general purpose, potential benefits, possible hazards and inconveniences of stress testing have been explained to my satisfaction and I have been given the opportunity to ask any questions that I have concerning the test.

I hereby consent to the performance of the test.

| | |
|---|---|
| _____ | _____ |
| Patient signature | Patient print name |
| _____ | _____ |
| Responsible physician signature | Responsible physician print name |

---

If a patient states that she is, or may be, pregnant or that she is breastfeeding, a radionuclide imaging study can only be performed after consulting with the RSO and the medical director. All benefits and risks must be weighed and discussed with the patient before proceeding with the procedure. The discussion should be documented in writing.

# PREPARATION FOR EXERCISE/STRESS PROTOCOLS

## *Stress Tc-99m-Agent (Tc-99m-Sestamibi or Tc-99m-Tetrofosmin) First*

- No coffee or caffeine-containing drinks or food can be ingested during the 12 h prior to the scheduled test.

- Patients are allowed to drink fruit juices, white milk, or water.
- Patients should be off theophylline-based medications for 48 h prior to the test. This should be done in consultation with the referring physicians

The reason for these instructions is that caffeine is a specific blocker of adenosine receptors and makes dipyridamole or adenosine infusion ineffective and will likely result in false-negative tests. (See Table 4-1.) It is not rare that a patient's exercise capacity is overestimated and they need to be switched to pharmacological stress. Therefore, as noted previously, it is advisable to give the same instruction about abstinence of caffeine-containing beverages and food to all scheduled patients.

- The patient should be nil per os (NPO) 4 h prior to stress. Patients with diabetes may eat a light meal (but no chocolate) and take their medications.
- Patients should continue their other medications unless directed otherwise by their physician.

### Rest Tc-99m-Agent (Tc-99m-Sestamibi or Tc-99m-Tetrofosmin) First

- The instructions are the same as for the "stress-first" procedure. However, the patients may eat a light breakfast or a light lunch if time permits before rest study. Patients should be NPO 4 h prior to stress.
- Patients should be off theophylline-based medications for 48 h following their physicians advice.

### Stress/Redistribution Tl-201

- Prior to the test the instructions are the same as for the "stress-first" procedure.
- Between the stress and redistribution part of the procedure, the patient may take liquids but no solid food. Caffeine is allowed after the stress portion. Diabetics may eat a light meal if needed.

The reason for this instruction is that ingestion of food after stress inhibits the redistribution of Tl-201 and defects may appear falsely fixed.

### Dual Isotope Rest-Thallium Stress-Tc-99m-Agent (Tc-99m-Sestamibi or Tc-99m-Tetrofosmin) Imaging

- The instructions are the same as for the "rest-first" procedure. The patients may eat a light breakfast or a light lunch if time permits before Rest study. Patients should be NPO 4 h prior to stress.

**Table 4-1**
**Caffeine-Containing Beverages, Food and Medications**
**that Compete with Adenosine Receptor Sites**

Beverages
    Coffee (including "decaffeinated" coffee)
    Tea
    Sodas (including regular, diet and "caffeine free" beverages)
    Chocolate drinks and chocolate products
Medications (partial list)
    Anacin®
    Exedrin®)
    Cold combination medication (Kolephrin)
    Goody's headache powder
    Keep Alert
    Midol®
    Amaphen
    Cafergot®
    Darvon®
    Fiorinal®
    Theophylline
    Theo-Dur®
    Oxtriphylline (Choledyl®)
    Aminophylline®

- Patients should be off theophylline-based medications for 48 h following their physicians advice.

# 5 Stress Procedures

In a well-run facility details of all procedures and policies are described in written protocols to ensure standardization and consistency of daily operations. Since no imaging facility operates under identical circumstances, protocols must be modified to meet specific needs. In order to meet standards for accreditation by the ICANL, for example, well-detailed "laboratory-specific protocols" play an important role (See Chapter 18 and on line: www.icanl.org). This chapter discusses:

- Indications and methodology
- Physical exercise testing
- Pharmacological stress testing

## PURPOSE OF STRESS PROCEDURES

Most stress procedures are performed in patients with symptoms of suspected or known ischemic heart disease . Patients must have stable symptoms or have been stabilized by therapy. The purpose of stress procedures is to provoke symptoms in a controlled and safe environment and thus aid in establishing the etiology of symptoms. Stress procedures must be performed under direct supervision by a physician.

### *Indications*

Appropriate clinical indications for stress testing are discussed in the "AHA/ACC 2002 Guideline Update for Exercise Testing," see: www.acc.org/clinical/guidelines/exercise/exercise.pdf. In brief they include:

1. Diagnosis of obstructive coronary artery disease.
2. Risk assessment and prognosis in patients with symptoms or known coronary artery disease.

From: *Contemporary Cardiology: Nuclear Cardiology, The Basics*
F. J. Th. Wackers, W. Bruni, and B. L. Zaret © Humana Press Inc., Totowa, NJ

## EXERCISE TESTING

Standard stress protocols are described in detail in "Updated imaging guidelines for nuclear cardiology procedures" *(1)* (on line: www.asnc.org; menu: library and resources: guidelines and standards).

Before exercise testing patient history must be obtained to identify any contraindications such as:

Recent acute myocardial infarction in the last four days
Unstable angina
Critical aortic stenosis
Congestive heart failure
Uncontrolled arrhythmias
Acute myocarditis/pericarditis
Aortic dissection.

It is important that patients understand the purpose and nature of the procedure. For example, in many instances the patient must recognize that the purpose of the test is to *reproduce symptoms* and that he/she must give his/her best effort; otherwise the test may be inconclusive.

A stress procedure, even an exercise ECG test, should never be performed without an IV in place. Cardiac emergencies may occur in apparently low-risk patients. Precious time may be lost if one has to establish IV access during cardiac resuscitation.

Perform a short and focused physical exam, which includes pulse, blood pressure, assessment of jugular vein distension, presence of edema, auscultation of the heart for gallops and heart murmur, and lung auscultation. Measure blood pressure with the patient in a standing position.

---

A good quality ECG is extremely important for diagnostic quality exercise testing. To ensure optimal quality ECG recordings during exercise without artifacts and interference , it is necessary to move the ECG electrodes from the conventional position on the extremities to the patient's trunk (see **Fig. 5-1**). The right and left upper extremity leads are moved closer to the sternum, whereas the lower extremity leads are moved to above the navel in the axillary line just below the rib cage.

---

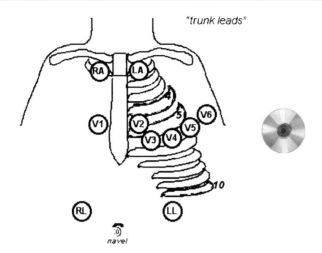

**Fig. 5-1.** Diagram of correct placement of radiotranslucent ECG electrodes during exercise. In order to reduce motion artifacts the extremity leads are moved from the limbs to the trunk.

---

**Measures that ensure optimal quality stress ECG tracings**
Proper skin preparation and lead placement
   Preparation of skin
   • Cleanse skin with alcohol, especially oily skin
   • Shave areas where electrodes are to be placed
   • Lightly abrade skin with scrubpads
   • Place electrode with the patient standing or sitting
Position electrodes correctly (see diagram)
   • Position Right Arm and Left Arm electrodes close to the sternum
Connect wires appropriately
   • Double check that right and left are not reversed

---

It should be appreciated that the modification in the extremity leads may result in a right axis shift and ST-segment changes in some patients. The exercise ECG should be compared to the rest *trunk* ECG and not the rest limb ECG.

**Causes for artifacts and noise on ECG and appropriate corrections**

Inadequate skin preparation
- Repeat preparation of skin and replace electrodes

Patient motion/tight grip on handle bar
- No excessive arm movements
- Hands should rest lightly on top of the handle bar

Inflation of blood pressure cuff
- Do not measure blood pressure while the ECG machine is printing

Lead reversal
- Replace leads according to color coding of the wires and according to schematic drawing

Trunk leads
- ECG obtained from trunk leads is slightly different compared to the conventional limb lead ECG

## *Methodology*

Although there are numerous graded exercise protocols, the Bruce protocol is the basis and most widely used method. For other protocols we refer to specialized texts on stress testing *(2,3)*.

**BRUCE PROTOCOL**

| Stage   | Speed | Incline | METs | Time |
|---------|-------|---------|------|------|
| Stage 1 | 1.7   | 10      | 4.6  | 3    |
| Stage 2 | 2.5   | 12      | 7.0  | 6    |
| Stage 3 | 3.4   | 14      | 10.1 | 9    |
| Stage 4 | 4.2   | 16      | 12.9 | 12   |
| Stage 5 | 5.0   | 18      | 15.0 | 15   |
| Stage 6 | 5.5   | 20      | 16.9 | 18   |

The treadmill should have a front rail. The patient may have the hands on top of the rail, but should not grip it too tightly. The patient should walk looking forward. An emergency stop button should be readily reached.

The treadmill is most commonly used in the United States because patients are more familiar with walking than with bicycling. However, in many other countries the upright stationary bicycle is used routinely

### Table 5-1
### Borg Scale of Perceived Exertion or Pain[a]

| | |
|---|---|
| 6 | |
| 7 | very, very light |
| 8 | |
| 9 | very light |
| 10 | |
| 11 | fairly light |
| 12 | |
| 13 | somewhat hard |
| 14 | |
| 15 | hard |
| 16 | |
| 17 | very hard |
| 18 | |
| 19 | very, very hard |
| 20 | |

[a]The Borg scale was developed based on the observation that young men can estimate their exercise heart rate in bpm by aligning a perceived level of exertion with a scale ranging from 6 to 20.

for physical stress testing. There are no real practical differences between the two forms of exercise for the purpose of diagnostic testing.

In older individuals and in those who have limited exercise capacity the Bruce protocol can be modified by two 3-min warm-up stages at 1.7 mph and 0 percent grade and 1.7 mph and 5 percent grade.

During the exercise protocol the patient should be monitored as follows:

- Record ECG, blood pressure, and heart rate at least at the end of every 3 min stage
- Continue to monitor ECG for changes and interrogate patients for symptoms (chest pain, lightheadedness, etc.).
- Consider using the BORG scale (see Table 5-1) as a reference to determine patient ability to continue physical exercise.
- Continue exercise until testing endpoint is reached. Optimally the patient will achieve the stage at which he/she perceives the work load as "17" or "18."

**Endpoints of exercise**

1. Reproduction of symptoms, angina
2. Marked fatigue and shortness of breath or wheezing
3. Achievement of at least 85% of age-predicted maximal heart rate (220–age). If patient is not symptomatic at this point, the stress test could continue
4. ≥ 2.5 mm asymptomatic horizontal/downsloping ST-segment depression
5. Leg cramps, claudication

**Absolute indications for terminating exercise test**

1. ST-segment elevation
2. Severe angina
3. Decrease of blood pressure (≥ 10 mmHg) with symptoms
4. Signs of poor peripheral perfusion: pallor, clammy skin, cyanosis
5. Central nervous system symptoms, such as ataxia, vertigo, confusion, gait problems
6. Serious arrhythmia: ventricular tachycardia, i.e., run ≥ 3 beats
7. Development of 2nd or 3rd degree AV block
8. Systolic blood pressure >220 mmHg or diastolic pressure >110 mmHg
9. Technical problems with monitoring vital parameters, including ECG
10. Patient's request

The most important and relevant clinical diagnostic end point is the reproduction of symptoms. If no symptoms occur, the attainment of target heart rate is only a general indication of the patient's effort. One should always attempt to achieve maximal effort with target heart rate as acceptable, but not necessarily ideal. If patient is unable to reach an adequate exercise endpoint, consider switching to vasodilator stress.

• Inject radiopharmaceutical when an exercise end point is attained
• After injection the patient should continue to walk for at least 2 more minutes.

Mark clock time of the injection of radiopharmaceutical relative to the start and end of exercise effort. The precise timing of the injection of the radiopharmaceutical is very important. It takes at least 4 min after the injection of radiopharmaceutical for the blood level to decrease to about 50% of injected dose *(4)*. Thus, the longer a patient continues to exercise after injection, the better the uptake in the heart reflects the exercise endpoint. However, in practice, it is usually not feasible to continue exercising for longer than 2 min after injection. The best approach is that the patient continues to exercise at the same maximal level for 1 min after injection, then to decrease the incline of the treadmill and speed as tolerated during the second minute.

After exercise, these procedures should be followed:

- Monitor blood pressure, heart rate, and ECG for 5 min
- Continue monitoring if chest pain or significant ECG changes persist
- Obtain 12-lead ECG after SPECT imaging is completed if necessary.
- Start imaging 15–30 min after termination of exercise.

## PHARMACOLOGICAL VASODILATION STRESS

Exercise stress is always the preferred stress modality for evaluating patients with known or suspected coronary artery disease. Pharmacological stress is indicated in patients who are unable to perform adequate physical stress due to:

- Musculoskeletal and neurologic conditions
- Peripheral vascular disease
- Pulmonary disease
- Left bundle branch block or paced rhythm
- Treatment with medications that blunt heart rate response (beta blockers, calcium channel blockers)
- Recent acute myocardial infarction 3–5 d

Standard stress protocols are described in detail in "Updated imaging guidelines for nuclear cardiology procedures" *(1)* (on line: www.asnc.org; menu: library and resources: guidelines and standards).

### DIPYRIDAMOLE

Patients with chronic obstructive pulmonary disease without bronchospasm usually tolerate infusion of dypiridamole well.

If active wheezing is present, the test should be switched to dobutamine infusion ( see below). One should be prepared for the development of high-degree AV-block. Patients with baseline first degree AV-block are at higher risk. In the latter patients one may consider switching to adenosine (relatively safer because of the short half life) or dobutamine.

Before dipyridamole vasodilator stress, the following should be obtained:

- Short patient history
- Focused physical examination to identify contraindications:
  Recent acute myocardial infarction
  Unstable angina
  Congestive heart failure
  Severe asthma and active wheezing
  Recent (< 24 h) use of caffeine-containing products (Table 4-1)

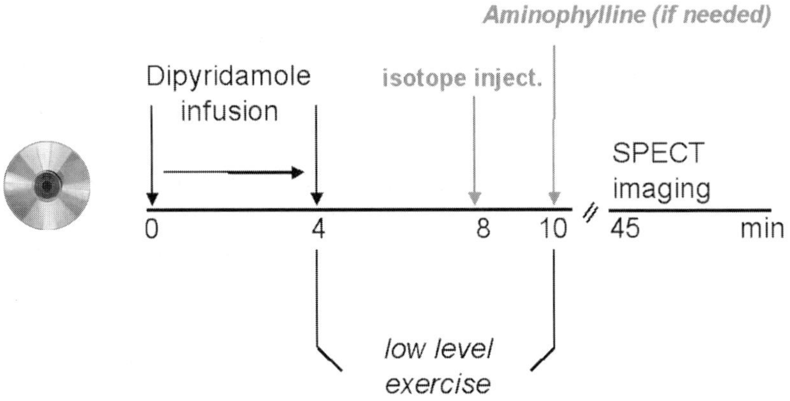

**Fig. 5-2.** Schematic representation of dipyridamole infusion protocol. After the infusion of dipyridamole is finished the patient may perform low level exercise.

- Explanation of procedure and possible side effects (It is important that the patient is warned about the side effects [Table 5-2] of dipyridamole infusion)
- Obtain IV access (for dipyridamole vasodilation one IV line is sufficient)
- Record baseline 12-lead ECG, heart rate, and blood pressure
- The dose of dipyridamole (5 mg/mL) is dependent on patient's weight Dipyridamole dose is diluted with normal saline to 40 mL

$$\frac{\text{Wt (kg)} \times 0.57 \text{ mg/kg}}{5 \text{ mg/mL}} = \text{mL of dipyridamole to be drawn up}$$

- Because of the long-acting effect of dipyridamole, the maximal dose generally administered is 60 mg
- Dipyridamole can be infused IV either by hand push over 4 min or by a motorized infusion pump

During vasodilator stress, the following procedures are important: (see **Fig. 5-2**)

- Record blood pressure, heart rate, and 12-lead ECG every minute. (If patient is able to walk, begin at slowest treadmill speed [Modified Bruce protocol stage 1] at 4 min after start of dipyridamole infusion.)
- Inject isotope at 8 min after start of infusion. The patient should continue walking for 2 min after radiopharmaceutical injection if at all feasible.
- At 10 min stop walking and monitor vital signs for 4–5 min into recovery.

- If side effects persist, administer aminophylline 75–125 mg IV over 2 min. (Avoid [if clinically safe] injecting aminophylline earlier than 2 min after injection of radiopharmaceutical as it may adversely affect the diagnostic yield of the test)

Aminophylline is a specific blocker of adenosine receptor sites. It is often needed to control symptoms caused by dipyridamole infusion. One should realize that the half-life of aminophylline is shorter than that of dipyridamole (40 min). Thus adverse effects may re-occur after approx 15 min and require another dose of aminophylline.

- Start imaging at 30–45 min after radiopharmaceutical injection if low-level exercise was performed, 45–60 min after radiopharmaceutical injection if no low-level exercise was performed.
- In patients with severe symptoms or ECG changes continue monitoring of vital signs and 12-lead ECG during imaging and after if necessary.

The performance of low-level exercise in combination with vasodi-lation has been shown to reduce unpleasant side effects, to decrease subdiaphragmatic radiotracer accumulation, and to increase heart rate moderately due to the minimal workload *(5,6)*.

## *Adenosine*

Before vasodilator stress, similar to the assessment prior to dipy-ridamole vasodilator stress, the following should be obtained:

- Short patient history
- Focused physical examination to identify contraindications:
    Recent acute myocardial infarction
    Unstable angina
    Congestive heart failure
    Severe asthma and active wheezing
    Greater than first degree heart block or sick sinus node syndrome
        without pacemaker
    Recent (<24 h) use of caffeine-containing products  (Table 4-1)
- Explanation of procedure and possible side effects (Table 5-2)
- Obtain IV access
- Record baseline 12-lead ECG, heart rate, and blood pressure
- Patients must have two separate IV lines or a short Y-connector attach-ment to prevent additional adenosine from being injected as a bolus during the injection of the radiopharmaceutical.
- Adenosine must be infused using a pump to ensure consistent dose administration. The dose of adenosine (a vial contains 3 mg/mL) is dependent on patient's weight:

**Table 5-2**
**Frequent Side Effects of Dipyridamole and Adenosine Infusion (% of Patients)**

|  | Dipyridamole (9) | Adenosine (10) |
|---|---|---|
| Cardiac |  |  |
| Fatal myocardial infarction | 0.05 | 0 |
| Nonfatal myocardial infarction | 0.05 | 0 |
| Chest pain | 19.7 | 57 |
| ST-T changes on ECG | 7.5 | 12 |
| Ventricular ectopy | 5.2 | ? |
| Tachycardia | 3.2 | ? |
| Hypotension | 4.6 | ? |
| Blood pressure instability | 1.6 | ? |
| Hypertension | 1.5 | ? |
| Atrio-ventricular block | 0 | 10 |
| Noncardiac |  |  |
| Headache | 12.2 | 35 |
| Dizziness | 11.8 | ? |
| Nausea | 4.6 | ? |
| Flushing | 3.4 | 29 |
| Pain (non specific) | 2.6 | ? |
| Dyspnea | 2.6 | 15 |
| Paraesthesia | 1.3 | ? |
| Fatigue | 1.2 | ? |
| Dyspepsia | 1.0 | ? |
| Acute bronchospasm | 0.15 | 0* |

*Patients with history of bronchospasm were excluded; ? not reported for adenosine

$$\frac{\text{Wt (kg)} \times 0.140 \text{ mg/kg/min} \times 6 \text{ min}}{3 \text{ mg}} = \text{mL of adenosine to be drawn up}$$

- Because of the short-acting effect of adenosine, there is no maximal dose limit
- If patient is able to walk, begin low-level exercise on treadmill without grade and at slowest speed
- When patient is comfortably walking, begin infusion of adenosine using a motorized infusion pump.

Adenosine should **Not** be injected by hand. It is impossible to mimic the steady slow flow of a motorized infusion pump. Because of the rapid action of adenosine, adverse effects are more likely to occur using hand push.

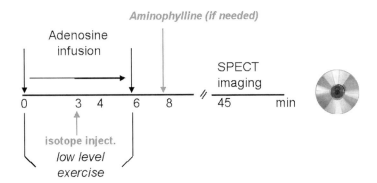

**Fig. 5-3.** Schematic representation of the long adenosine infusion protocol. During the infusion of adenosine the patient may perform low level exercise.

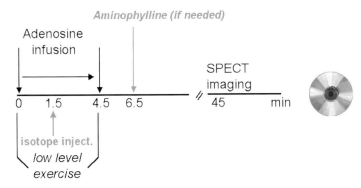

**Fig. 5-4.** Schematic representation of the short adenosine infusion protocol. During the infusion of adenosine the patient may perform low level exercise.

There are two commonly used adenosine infusion protocols: the conventional **long protocol (Fig. 5-3)** and the **short protocol (Fig. 5-4)**. Conventional protocol is as follows:

- Adenosine is infused over a 6-min period
- The radiopharmaceutical is injected during the third minute of infusion. Infusion is then continued for an additional 3 min

Because of the rapid onset of vasodilation of adenosine, a **shortened protocol** has become popular *(7,8)*.

- The radiopharmaceutical is injected at 1.5 min into infusion. The infusion is then continued for an additional 3 min (i.e., a total 4.5-min infusion).

During vasodilator stress, follow these procedures:

- Record blood pressure, heart rate, and 12-lead ECG every minute

- Record occurrence of symptoms (chest pain, lightheadedness, SOB, nausea, etc.)
- Mark clock time of the injection of radiopharmaceutical relative to the start and end of dipyridamole or adenosine infusion.
- After injection of the radiopharmaceutical, the infusion continues for 3 min and the patient continues to walk
- The patient stops walking when the infusion is stopped.

After vasodilator stress, follow these procedures:

- Monitor blood pressure, heart rate, and ECG for 5 min after the completion of infusion
- Continue clinical monitoring if chest pain or significant ECG changes persist
- Give aminophylline (75–125 mg IV over 2–3 min) when indicated for symptoms. If at all clinically possible, this should be delayed until at least 2 min after radiopharmaceutical injection.
- Obtain 12-lead ECG after SPECT imaging is completed if necessary.
- Start imaging 30–45 min after radiopharmaceutical injection

If necessary (in patients with symptoms or ECG changes [Table 5-2]) continue monitoring vital signs and 12-lead ECG during and after completion of imaging.

## PHARMACOLOGIC ADRENERGIC STRESS

Pharmacological adrenergic stress (with dobutamine) (Fig. 5-5) is indicated in patients who cannot undergo physical exercise stress and have contraindications to pharmacological vasodilator stress.

Standard stress protocols are described in detail in "Updated imaging guidelines for nuclear cardiology procedures" *(1)* (on line: www.asnc.org; menu: library and resources: guidelines and standards).

### *Dobutamine*

In general, the patient population that requires dobutamine stress is a more selected and sicker population. It is important that the patient is warned about possible side effects of dobutamine infusion. The increase in heart rate and palpitations are often experienced as unpleasant (see Table 5-3).

Before adrenergic stress, similar to the assessment prior to exercise testing, the following should be obtained:

- Short patient history
- Focused physical examination to identify contraindications:
    Acute myocardial infarction within prior 5 d
    Unstable angina

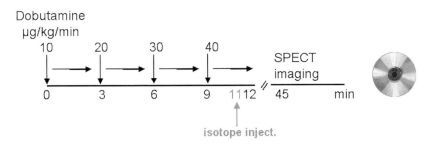

**Fig. 5-5.** Schematic representation of dobutamine infusion protocol.

**Table 5-3**
**Frequent Side Effects of Intravenous Dobutamine** *(11)*

| Cardiac | % of patients |
|---|---|
| Fatal myocardial infarction | 0 |
| Nonfatal myocardial infarction | 0 |
| Chest pain | 31 |
| ST-T changes on ECG | 50 |
| Ventricular ectopy | 43 |
| Tachycardia | 1.4 |
| Hypotension | 0 |
| Hypertension | 1.4 |
| AV block | 0.6 |
| Noncardiac | |
| Headache | 14 |
| Dizziness | 4 |
| Nausea | 9 |
| Flushing | 14 |
| Pain (nonspecific) | 7 |
| Dyspnea | 14 |
| Paraesthesia | 12 |

    Congestive heart failure
    Critical aortic stenosis
    Known supraventricular or ventricular tachycardia
    Uncontrolled hypertension
    Beta blocking medication
- Explanation of procedure and possible side effects (Table 5-3).
- Patients must have two separate IV lines or a short Y-connector attachment to prevent additional dobutamine from being injected as a bolus during the injection of the radiopharmaceutical.
- Record baseline 12-lead ECG, heart rate, and blood pressure.

During adrenergic stress, the following procedures are important:

- The dose of dobutamine is dependent on patient weight and the time into the protocol.
- Dobutamine must be infused using a motorized pump to allow for variable infusion rates.
- Dobutamine is infused starting at $10\,\mu g/kg/min$, increasing the dose every 3 min: $20\,\mu g/kg/min$, $30\,\mu g/kg/min$, up to a maximum of $40\,\mu g/kg/min$.
- Record blood pressure, heart rate, and 12-lead ECG every minute
- Monitor occurrence of symptoms (chest pain, lightheadedness, shortness of breath, nausea, etc.) and arrhythmias.
- Monitor vital signs for 4–5 min into recovery: side effects should subside within 5 min of completion of infusion. Continue monitoring or obtain 12-lead ECG postimaging if necessary.
- In some laboratories atropine (0.5–2 mg IV) may be given if the target heart rate has not been attained at maximal dobutamine dose.
- Inject radiopharmaceutical at 11 min of protocol or at target heart rate
- Mark clock time of the injection of radiopharmaceutical relative to the start and end of dobutamine infusion.
- Start imaging 30–45 min after radiopharmaceutical injection.

If necessary (in patients with symptoms or ECG changes) continue monitoring vital signs and 12-lead ECG during and after completion of imaging.

After adrenergic stress, follow these procedures:

- Monitor blood pressure, heart rate, and ECG for 5 min after the completion of infusion.
- Continue clinical monitoring if chest pain or significant ECG changes persist.
- Give metoprolol (5–15 mg IV over 2–3 min) when indicated for symptoms. If at all clinically possible, this should be delayed until at least 2 min after radiopharmaceutical injection.
- Obtain, if necessary, follow-up 12-lead ECG after SPECT imaging is completed.

## STRESS PROTOCOL WORKSHEETS

Worksheets are useful for documentation of the details of a stress test, the patient's symptoms, drug given, etc. Below are sample worksheets for pharmacological vasodilator stress used in our laboratory.

## CARDIAC EXERCISE LABORATORY
## DIPYRIDAMOLE PROTOCOL

Date:_____

Name:_____     Unit Number:_____

Wt_____ kg
Ht_____cm

Dipyridamole infused at 0.142 mg/kg/min for 4 min, for a total of 0.57 mg/kg

1. _____kg X 0.57 mg/kg =_____total mg infused
2. _____total mg infused/4 min = _____mg/min infused
3. _____total mg infused/5 =_____mL of Dipyridamole to be drawn up in a 60 mL syringe
4. Reconstitute Dipyridamole with NaCl = 40 ml
5. Manually push 10 mL/min over the next 4 minutes
6. Isotope injected at 8 min
7. BP and 12 Lead ECG every minute

Baseline H.R._____ B.P. _____

| Time from start EFFECTS of infusion | H.R. | B.P. | COMMENTS/SIDE |
|---|---|---|---|
| 1 | | | |
| 2 | | | |
| 3 | | | |
| 4 | | | |
| 5 | | | |
| 6 | | | |
| 7 | | | |
| Isotope injected 8 | | | |
| 9 | | | |
| 10 | | | |

Side Effects:

Onset_____ min                          Duration
_____min

Aminophylline amount_____ mg     Time inj._____ Min

CARDIAC EXERCISE LABORATORY
6 MINUTE ADENOSINE PROTOCOL

Date:_____

1. 2 IV's or Y connector required
2. Infusion over 6 minutes via pump
3. Radioisotope injected at 3 minutes
4. Blood pressure and 12 lead ECG every min.

Name:_____          Unit Number:_____

Wt_____ kg
Ht_____cm

Adenosine infused:_____kg X 0.140 mg/kg/min/3 mg = _____mL/min =
Infusion rate/min

1. _____ mL/min (infusion rate) X 6 =_____total mls infused over 6 min
2. _____total ml infused + 3 ml for tubing dead space = _____ total
Adenosine to be drawn up
3. Place the total mls obtained from #2 in a 30 ml syringe
( If this number > 30 ml, use a 60 mL syringe )
4. DO NOT DILUTE USING GRAESBY PUMP.
5. If patient weighs more than 310 lbs use Bolus Mode on Graesby pump

Baseline H.R._____ B.P. _____

| Time from start EFFECTS of infusion | H.R. | B.P. | COMMENTS/SIDE |
|---|---|---|---|
| 1 | | | |
| 2 | | | |
| Isotope inj. 3 | | | |
| 4 | | | |
| 5 | | | |
| Stop Adeno 6 | | | |
| 7 | | | |

*Total mLs. Infused over 6 min (#1) _____ X 3mg = _____mg infused
Side Effects:
Onset_____ min                          Duration
_____min
Aminophylline amount_____ mg      Time inj._____ Min

# SELECTED BIBLIOGRAPHY

1. DePuey GE, Garcia EV (2001). Updated imaging guidelines for nuclear cardiology procedures, *Part I. J Nucl Cardiol* 8:G1–58.
2. Ellestad MH (ed) (1995). Stress testing, principles and practice, 4th edition, FA Davis Co.
3. Froelicher VF (2000). Exercise and the Heart, 4th edition, WB Saunders Co.
4. Wackers FJTh. Myocardial perfusion imaging, Chapter 15 in: Sandler MP, Coleman RE, Patton JA, Wackers FJTh, Gottschalk A (eds) (2003). Diagnostic Nuclear Medicine, Fourth Edition, Lippincott Williams & Wilkins, Philadelphia, PA.
5. Penell DJ , Maurogeni S, Forbat SM, et al. (1995). Adenosine combined with dynamic exercise for myocardial perfusion imaging. *J Am Coll Cardiol* 25:1300–1309.
6. Samady H, Wackers FJTh, Joska TM, Zaret BL, Jain D (2002). Pharmacologic stress perfusion imaging with adenosine:role of simultaneous low-level treadmill exercise. *J Nucl Cardiol* 9:188–196.
7. Treuth MG, Reyes GA, He ZX, Cwajg E, Mahamarian JJ, Verani MS (2001). Tolerance and diagnostic accuracy of an abbreviated adenosine infusion for myocardial scintigraphy: A randomized, prospective study. *J Nucl Cardiol* 8:548–554.
8. O'Keefe JH, Bateman TM, Handlin LR, Barnhart CS (1995). Four- versus 6-minute protocol for adenosine thallium-201 single photon emission computed tomography imaging. *Am Heart J* 129:482–487.
9. Ranhosky A, Rawson J (1990). The safety of intravenous dipyridamole thallium myocardial perfusion imaging. *Circulation* 81:1205.
10. Verani MS, Mahmarian JJ, Hixson JB, et al. (1990). Diagnosis of coronary artery disease by controlled coronary vasodilation with adenosine and thallium-201 scintigraphy in patients unable to exercise. *Circulation* 82:80.
11. Hays JT, Mahmarian JJ, Cochran AJ, et al. (1993). Dobutamine thallium-201 tomography for evaluating patients with suspected coronary artery disease unable to undergo exercise or vasodilator pharmacologic stress testing. *J Am Coll Cardiol* 21:1583.

# 6   SPECT Myocardial Perfusion Imaging Acquisition and Processing Protocols

In view of the variety of gamma camera systems that are commercially available, it is difficult to incorporate every acquisition/acquisition parameter adequately into a few simple charts. Single-headed systems have different acquisition parameters than triple-headed systems, and both are different from dual-headed systems. One must also consider the radiopharmaceutical(s) and imaging protocols one employed. Acquisition parameters will vary depending on these variables.

This chapter highlights:

- Acquisition parameters
- Processing parameters

---

Once the purchase of a gamma camera has been made, it is advisable that a professional application specialist visit the laboratory to train the technical staff in applying the vendor-recommended acquisition and processing protocols. This is crucial for optimal results.

Nuclear cardiology tests are to be performed under general physician supervision. That is, the medical director is responsible on an ongoing basis for the training of nonphysician personnel who actually perform the diagnostic procedures, for protocols and policies, and for the appropriate maintenance of necessary equipment and supplies.

All acquisition parameters listed in Table 6-1 are based on the "Updated imaging guidelines for nuclear cardiology procedures" *(1)* (on line: www.asnc.org; menu: library and resources: guidelines and stan-

From: *Contemporary Cardiology: Nuclear Cardiology, The Basics*
F. J. Th. Wackers, W. Bruni, and B. L. Zaret © Humana Press Inc., Totowa, NJ

**Table 6-1**
**Acquisition Parameters**

|  | *Tc-99m* | *Tl-201* |
|---|---|---|
| Dose | 10–30 mCi | 3.5–4.5 mCi |
| Collimator | High resolution | Low energy all-purpose |
|  | Matrix parallel hole | parallel hole |
|  | 64 × 64 | 64 × 64 |
|  | Peak 140 keV, | 78 keV 30% centered |
|  | 20% centered |  |
| Gating | 8 or 16 frames/cycle | 8 frames/cycle |
| No. of projections | 64 | 32 |
| Orbit | 180° | 180° |
| Orbit type | Circular | Circular |
| Acquisition type | Step and shoot/continuous | Step and shoot /continuous |
| Pixel size | 6.4 ± 0.2 mm | 6.4 ± 0.2 mm |
| Time/projection | 25 s for low doses | 40 s (at least) |
|  | 20 s for high doses |  |
| Attenuation | Different for different | Different for different |
| correction | vendors | vendors |

dards). Additional information on accepted standards for performing myocardial perfusion imaging can be found in the Society of Nuclear Medicine Procedure Guidelines for Myocardial Perfusion Imaging (on line: www.snm.org/policy/new_guidelines_1. html).

A review of **clinical indications** for myocardial perfusion imaging can be found on line: www.acc.org/clinical/radio/57252.pdf and in: Guidelines for clinical use of cardiac radionuclide imaging 2 (these Guidelines are currently under revision).

The time interval from injection of radiopharmaceutical to the start of imaging is:

|  | Exercise | PharmStress | Rest |
|---|---|---|---|
| T1-201 | 10 min | 10 min | 30 min |
| Tc-99m-agent | 15 min | 45 min | 45 min |

## ACQUISITION PARAMETERS

The acquisition parameters are listed in Table 6-1. In this and following tables doses are given in mCi. Note: 1 mCi = 37 MBq. The following subsections are comments on the individual parameters listed.

### *Dose*

It is prudent to institute weight criteria for the choice of imaging agents, Tl-201 or Tc-99m-agent, and imaging protocols, one-day or two-

**Table 6-2**
**Suggested Weight Limits for**
**Selecting Appropriate Imaging Agent and Protocols**

| Male | Female | Agent/Protocol |
|------|--------|----------------|
| ≤ 225 lb (102 kg) | ≤ 150 lb (68 kg) | T-201 or Tc-99m agent *1-day or 2-day protocol* |
| 226–275 lb (103–124 kg) | 151–175 lb (69–79 kg) | only Tc-99m agent *1-day or 2-day protocol* |
| ≥ 276 lb (125 kg) | ≥ 176 lb (80 kg) | only Tc-99m agent *only 2-day protocol* |

day protocols (Table 6-2). In obese patients imaging with Tc-99m-agent is preferred over imaging with Tl-201, and in very obese patients a two-day imaging protocol is preferred over the one-day imaging protocol. When a patient is markedly obese, even the standard dose of 25 mCi per day of a Tc-99-agent may not be adequate. In these obese patients the dose can be adjusted according to the patient's weight. It is advisable to check with the RSO about such upward dose adjustments. Table 6-3 shows examples of dose adjustment on the basis of weight used in our laboratory. The weight limits are based on practical experience. Since in females more of the increased weight is generally in the upper body, the adjusted doses are higher in females than in males.

*Note: In addition to adjusting the dose, one may also increase acquisition time per stop to improve the quality of study.*

## DEVIATION FROM STANDARD RADIOPHARMACEUTICAL DOSING

It is recommended that all deviations from the standard dosing are discussed with the RSO and/or the medical director. If it is necessary to make higher dose adjustments due to obesity, the deviation should be approved by the RSO as appropriate.

Doses for pediatric patients should also be discussed with the RSO.

A patient under 18 years of age would have the dose adjusted with the following formula.

$$\frac{\text{Patient weight in lb}}{150 \text{ lb}} \times \text{standard dose (mCi)} = \text{pediatric dose (mCi)}$$

## *Collimator*

Low-energy high-resolution collimators (LEHR) provide better resolution but reduced sensitivity; therefore, they are usually used with the

**Table 6-3**
**Suggested Dose Adjustments of Tl-201**
**and Tc-99m-Labeled Agents on the Basis of Weight**

| *Tl-201* | *Male mCi* | *Female mCi* |
|---|---|---|
| Weight | | |
| 125–150 lb (56–68 kg) | 3.0 | 4.0 |
| 151–175 lb (69–79 kg) | 3.5 | 4.5* |
| 176–200 lb (80–90 kg) | 4.0 | 4.5* |
| 201–225 lb (91–102 kg) | 4.5 | 4.5* |
| ≥ 226 lb (103 kg) | 4.5* | 4.5* |
| or | | |
| Chest circumference | | |
| ≤ 44 in (112 cm) | 3.5 | |
| 45–48 in (113–122 cm) | 4.0 | |
| > 48 in (123 cm) | 4.5* | |
| *Tc-99-labeled agents (2-day protocol, daily dose)* | | |
| Weight | | |
| 175–200 lb (79–90 kg) | 25 | 30 |
| 201–250 lb (91–113 kg) | 25 | 30 |
| 251–275 lb (114–124 kg) | 25 | 35* |
| 276–300 lb (125–136 kg) | 30 | 40* |
| 301–325 lb (137–147 kg) | 35* | 40* |
| 326–350 lb (148–159 kg) | 40* | 45* |

*It may be advisable to increase acquisition time per stop as well

Tc-99m agents, which yield higher count rates. Low-energy all-purpose (LEAP) collimators provide more sensitivity and are routinely used to imagine Tl-201.

When performing dual-isotope studies, one should use the same collimator for both the rest Tl-201 and the stress Tc-99m study. The high-resolution collimator is preferred in this circumstance.

## *Matrix*

A 64 × 64 matrix is standard for SPECT imaging. A 128 × 128 matrix also can be used; however, this substantially increases the required computer disk storage space. In addition, processing time will increase significantly.

## *ECG Gating*

### CHEST ELECTRODES

For ECG gating the computer should receive a clear R-wave signal. Usually three electrodes are used: right and left subclavicular and one on the lateral lower chest (either right or left). If this conventional electrode placement does not work, move the electrodes around to a position that results in a more distinct R-wave. (Make sure that in patients with abnormal ECG or peaked T waves no double signal is detected.)

### NUMBERING OF FRAMES PER R-R CYCLE

Eight frames/cycle is standard practice and gives adequate results. Because of limited temporal resolution, left ventricular ejection fraction (LVEF) is systematically underestimated. The lower limit of normal for 8-frame LVEF is 0.45. To obtain a more accurate LVEF SPECT, acquisition with 16 frames/cycle is required. A disadvantage is that acquisition of 16-frames/cycle gated SPECT studies requires considerably more hard drive space, archiving space, and fast(er) computer for processing.

## *Number of Projections*

When performing high-resolution studies with Tc-99m perfusion agents, it is recommended acquiring 64 projections over a 180° arc. Lower-resolution studies acquired with Tl-201 need only 32 projections.

It should be noted that the number of recommended projections might vary from this depending on the manufacturer and the number of camera heads on the system.

## *Orbit*

A circular orbit is the most commonly used orbit. This orbit maintains the camera head at a fixed distance from the patient. Noncircular or elliptical orbits should be used with caution, because they may create artifacts due to varying depth resolution resulting from varying "detector–heart" distance.

In the ASNC Guidelines for cardiac SPECT image acquisition with 180° orbits is recommended (45° RAO to 45° LPO), a 360° orbit is optional *(1)*. The reason for this is that a 180° orbit avoids the degrading effects of scatter and attenuation from the posterior projections. This is especially relevant when low-energy Tl-201 imaging is performed. However, using Tc-99m agents, a 180° acquisition orbit in some patients may create image distortion and inhomogeneity in the most apical short axis slices. In our experience, these artifacts can be avoided by acquiring SPECT images with a 360° orbit *(3)*.

## Acquisition Mode

The step-and-shoot acquisition mode is most commonly used and is standard because it allows for ECG-gated acquisition. During the step-and-shoot mode, the camera moves to a position, stops, and acquires an image for a set time and then moves on to the next angle. No image acquisition occurs during the motion of the camera. In continuous acquisition mode the camera acquires image data constantly while moving slowly along the orbit. Currently, this acquisition mode may not allow for ECG-gated acquisition on some systems. Some systems now have a continuous step-and-shoot mode that provides the benefits of both acquisition types

## Pixel Size

A 6.4 ± 0.2-mm pixel size for a 64 × 64 matrix provides adequate image resolution and is considered standard.

## Time Per Projection

The time per projection must be long enough to obtain sufficient counts for producing images of optimal quality. Reducing the time per projection too much will result in low count density and suboptimal image quality. The time per projection depends on the number of projections acquired over the orbit. For Tl-201 SPECT the time per stop should be at least 40 s. However, depending on count density and patient weight, it may have to be as long as 60 s. The limiting factor is the amount of time that one can expect a patient to lie immobile on the imaging table. Generally, total imaging time should not be much longer than 20 min. The significant advantage of multiheaded camera systems is that image data are acquired simultaneously at different angles, thus maximizing image quality (=counts) within a limited time.

## Attenuation Correction

At the present time each vendor uses different technology and methodology for nonuniform tissue attenuation correction. Transmission data are acquired using a variety of approaches (i.e., moving rods containing transmission sources or X-ray CT). Although it is recognized that SPECT images should not only be corrected for nonuniform tissue attenuation, but also for scatter and depth-dependent resolution, not all vendors apply all three corrections. Some methods allow for simultaneous acquisition of the transmission (attenuation) and emission (perfusion) data. If this is feasible, the total acquisition time is not substantially longer and is thus time efficient. Other vendors require the transmission data to be acquired either after or before acquisition of emission data. The latter approach may add considerably to the total acquisition time of a study. Because

### Table 6-4
### Processing Parameters

| | |
|---|---|
| Filtering | Filtered back projection is standard; cutoffs and frequencies are vendor dependent. |
| Motion correction | After applying correction program, slices must be evaluated for motion artifacts. Many programs are not adequate. |
| Reconstruction | Reorienting of data into vertical and horizontal long-axis and short-axis planes. |
| Slice alignment | Aligning stress slices to the corresponding rest slices. |
| Normalizing slices | Scaling of images so the heart is visualized optimally. |
| Attenuation correction | Acquisition of transmission mask for non-uniform tissue attenuation correction. Different approaches are used by each vendor. |
| Quantification | Plot of count density of each slice. |
| Normal database | Allows extent and severity of defect to be calculated. |
| Left ventricular ejection fraction | Automated estimate of myocardial systolic function. |
| Left ventricular volume | The same software that provides ejection fraction also estimates left ventricular end diastolic and end systolic volumes. |
| Archiving | Raw and processed data. |

each camera system uses different techniques to perform SPECT attenuation correction, it is very important to refer and adhere to optimized acquisition parameters defined by the manufacturer. An applications specialist should visit the imaging facility and train the technical staff on site on proper use of attenuation correction. Attenuation correction technology is very different from standard emission myocardial perfusion imaging.

## PROCESSING PARAMETERS

The processing parameters are listed in Table 6-4. The following subsections are comments on the individual parameters listed.

### *Filtering*

The purpose of image filters is to remove noise and blur before and after back projection of raw SPECT data. The standard filter for SPECT imaging is the Butterworth filter. The optimal order and cut-off of this

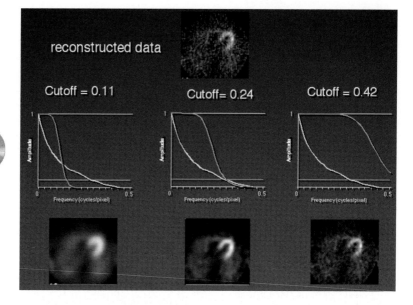

**Fig. 6-1.** The effect of different cut-offs for a low-pass Butterworth filter is well illustrated in this figure. The preferred cutoff for this particular image is 0.24. A lower low cutoff, e.g., 0.11, results in a markedly blurred image with loss of detail. A higher cutoff , e.g., 0.42, results in a noisy image. One should experiment with various filter cutoffs using equipment in the laboratory and study their the differential effect on image quality.

filter is different for each vendor. Excellent reviews about filters are available by Zubal *(4)* and Hanson *(5–7)*.

### *Motion Correction*

Motion on SPECT studies can be detected in a number of ways. Some systems provide the option of displaying a "sinogram." Breaks or irregularities in the sinogram indicate motion. This display method is not always easy to interpret. Sinograms do not show horizontal motion, but only vertical or Y-axis motion. A simple, and more commonly used method for detecting patient motion, involves inspection of the cine display of all planar projection images, i.e., rotating images. This simple method allows for the detection of both X-axis and Y-axis motion.

If motion is detected, a motion-correction program can be applied. Each vendor may have a slightly different approach to motion correction. One should consult with the vendor for instructions on how to run the program. Motion-corrected cine should be viewed to determine if the motion was corrected. Under certain conditions the correction program may not work and in some instances it may create even worse artifacts. If the program does not correct motion adequately, the entire imaging

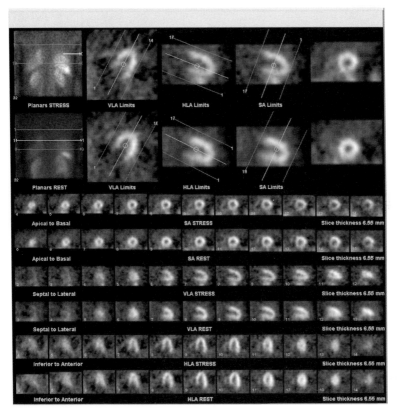

**Fig. 6-2.** Computer screen display of the reorientation of reconstructed tomographic slices to the anatomical axis of the heart. The boundaries of the window of reconstruction are indicated by red lines. The green lines indicate the angles of tomographic slicing for the vertical long axis (VLA), horizontal long axis (HLA), and the short axis (SA).

study should be repeated. Even if it appears that the program has corrected the motion on cine display, the reconstructed slices should be inspected for motion artifacts. Typical motion artifacts are gaps at the apex of the long-axis slices and breaks in the short axis slices to make them look disjointed. See Chapter 14 for examples.

Note that some motion-correction programs are very specific and work only on certain types of acquisition data. For instance, not all programs are capable of correcting ECG-gated image data and some correct only 180° acquisition data and not 360° acquisition data.

## Reconstruction

This step reorients the data to the 3 axes of the patient's heart. Horizontal long axis, vertical long axis, and short axis slices are created. It is crucial that the stress and rest slices be reconstructed identically in order for the same segments to be compared.

## Slice Alignment

The stress and rest slices must be aligned or matched. The first apical slice of the stress study must match the first apical slice of the rest study and continue on through to the last basal slice. If the slices are misaligned, the study may be misinterpreted.

## Normalizing Slices

This step is particularly important when imaging with the Tc-99m agents. Often, particularly after pharmacological stress, the liver or bowel, and not the heart, are the organs with the most intense activity. The heart is then hardly visible unless images are scaled properly to increase the intensity of the heart image.

## Attenuation Correction

Most vendors provide the option of applying attenuation correction to myocardial perfusion images. If used, it is recommended that the myocardial perfusion data be processed first without attenuation correction and then reprocessed with attenuation correction. While attenuation corrected images are often very helpful, the technology is demanding (8). Attenuation corrected images may at times contain artifacts or overcorrections. The interpreter must have the ability to take these into account during image analysis. Therefore, it is often helpful to *inspect both the attenuation corrected and the uncorrected images*. Ask the vendor about quality-assurance criteria for their specific attenuation-correction device/methodology.

## Quantification

The relative distribution of a radiopharmaceutical in reconstructed myocardial slices can be quantified using a number of commercially available software packages. Regional relative radiotracer uptake is compared to regional lower limits of normal uptake. For accurate and reproducible quantitative results, it is important that the apical and basal slices are chosen appropriately in accordance with the vendor's manual.

## Normal Database

A normal database is generated from images of normal subjects with low (<3%) likelihood of coronary artery disease, based on age, gender, absence of symptoms and risk factors, and normal exercise ECG. From the relative count distribution on images of these normal subjects, a

## SPECT MYOCARDIAL PERFUSION WORKSHEET

Patient Name _____

       Unit # _____        Weight _____        Height _____

       Floor _____        Chest _____        Cup_____

   One Day ☐        Two Day ☐        Camera _____

| STRESS IMAGING | REST IMAGING |
|---|---|
| Date _____ | Date _____ |
| ☐ Exercise    ☐ Adenosine / ☐ Aden/Ex | ☐ Rest    ☐ Redist |
| Other _____ | |
| MIBI _____ mCi    Initials: ____ | MIBI _____ mCi    Initials: ____ |
| Tl-201 _____ mCi | Tl-201 _____ mCi |
| Other _____    _____ mCi | Other _____    _____ mCi |
| Inject Time: _____ | Inject Time: _____ |
| TT: _____ | TT: _____ |
| _____ SPECT Time | _____ SPECT Time |
| _____ Radius | _____ Radius |
| _____ Table Height | _____ Table Height |
| _____ sec/stop | _____ sec/stop |
| _____ GATED | _____ GATED |
| PLANARS    5 min | PLANARS    5 min |
| TIME    Angle | TIME    Angle |
| _____ LATS    (0)_____ | _____ LATS    (0)_____ |
| _____ LATD    (90)_____ | _____ LATD    (90)_____ |
| **DEFECT SCORE** | **DEFECT SCORE** |
| __ __ __ __ __ | __ __ __ __ __ |
| Api   Mid   Bas   Apx   Gbl | Api   Mid   Bas   Apx   Gbl |
| WLCQ EF: _____ | WLCQ EF: _____ |
| QGS (opt.): _____ | QGS (opt.): _____ |
| Technologist _____ | Technologist _____ |

COMMENTS:

lower limit of normal count distribution, i.e., mean minus two standard deviations, can be derived.

## *Left Ventricular Ejection Fraction*

A number of commercially available software packages exist for calculation of left ventricular ejection fraction (LVEF) from ECG-gated SPECT images. Accurate assessment of LVEF depends on stable heart rate, adequate counts, and good image quality. One has the option of acquiring a gated SPECT study with either 16 or 8 frames per RR-cycle. The lower limit of normal LVEF using a 16-frame study is higher ( 0.50) than for a 8-frame study (0.45) *(9)*. Intense noncardiac activity and small hearts may render calculation of LVEF inaccurate *(10)*.

## *Left Ventricular Volumes*

Left ventricular volumes are estimated from the endocardial boundaries used to calculate ejection fraction. End diastolic and end systolic volumes derived from ECG-gated SPECT studies often appear to be relatively small. Nevertheless, several studies have shown good correlations with volumes derived by other modalities *(11)*.

## *Archiving*

All raw image data should be archived daily. It is recommended processed and quantified data be archived for comparison with future studies.

## TECHNOLOGIST WORKSHEETS

Worksheets are useful for documentation of the details of an imaging procedure, such as patient body habitus, dose, time of injection, time of imaging, and other details. A sample of the worksheet for myocardial perfusion imaging used in our laboratory is given on page 71.

## SELECTED BIBLIOGRAPHY

1. DePuey GE, Garcia EV (2001). Updated imaging guidelines for nuclear cardiology procedures, Part I. *J Nucl Cardiol* 8:G1–58.
2. ACC/AHA Task Force (1995). Guidelines for clinical use of cardiac radionuclide imaging. *J Am Coll Cardiol* 25:521–547.
3. Liu YH, Lam PT, Sinusa AJ, Wackers FJ. (2001). Differential effect of 180° and 360° acquisition orbits in the accuracy of SPECT imaging: quantitative evaluation in phantoms. *J Nucl Med* 43:1115–1124.
4. Zubal IG, Wisniewski G (1997). Understanding Fourier space and filter selection. *J Nucl Cardiol* 4:234–243.
5. Hanson CL (2002). Digital image processing for clinicians, part I. Basics of image formation. *J Nucl Cardiol* 9:343–349.
6. Hanson CL (2002). Digital image processing for clinicians, part II. Filtering. *J Nucl Cardiol* 9:429–437.
7. Hanson CL (2002). Digital image processing for clinicians, part III. SPECT reconstruction. *J Nucl Cardiol* 9:542–549.
8. Hendel RC, Corbett JR, Cullom J, DePuey EG, Garcia EV (2002). The value and practice of attenuation correction for myocardial perfusion imaging: a joint position statement from the American Society of Nuclear Cardiology. *J Nucl Cardiol* 9:135–143.
9. Germano G, Kiat H, Kavanagh PB, et al. (1995). Automatic quantification of ejection fraction from gated myocardial perfusion SPECT. *J Nucl Med* 36:2138–2147.
10. Vallejo E, Dione DP, Sinusas AJ, Wackers FJTh (2000). Assessment of left ventricular ejection fraction with quantitative gated SPECT: accuracy and correlation with first-pass radionuclide angiography. *J Nucl Cardiol* 7:461–470.
11. Iskandrian AE, Germano G, Van Decker W, et al. (1998). Validation of left ventricular volume measurements by gated SPECT 99m Tc-labeled sestamibi imaging. *J Nucl Cardiol* 5:574–578.

# 7
# Planar Myocardial Perfusion Imaging Acquisition and Processing Protocols

Although the use of planar myocardial perfusion imaging has decreased drastically in the last 10 yr, some patients can be imaged *only* using the planar technique. These are patients with claustrophobia, patients who are too heavy for the SPECT imaging table, and patients who cannot remain immobile on the imaging table for an extended period of time.

When performed with optimal technique and attention to details, planar imaging can result in good quality visualization of regional myocardial perfusion and diagnostic information that approaches that of SPECT imaging. A substantial portion of the literature on radionuclide myocardial perfusion imaging until the early 1990s was based on planar imaging.

All acquisition parameters listed in the following tables are based on the "Updated imaging guidelines for nuclear cardiology procedures" *(1)* (on line: www.asnc.org; menu: library and resources: guidelines and standards). **Clinical indications** for nuclear cardiology imaging can be found on line: www.acc.org/clinical/radio/57252.pdf, Guidelines for clinical use of cardiac radionuclide imaging *(2)*. (These guidelines are presently under revision.)

## PLANAR MYOCARDIAL PERFUSION IMAGING

Table 7-1 lists the acquisition parameters for planar myocardial perfusion imaging. The accompanying box details the factors required for optimal quality imaging.

From: *Contemporary Cardiology: Nuclear Cardiology, The Basics*
F. J. Th. Wackers, W. Bruni, and B. L. Zaret © Humana Press Inc., Totowa, NJ

**Table 7-1**
**Acquisition Parameters**

|              | *Tc-99m*                       | *Tl-201*                       |
|--------------|--------------------------------|--------------------------------|
| Dose         | 10–30 mCi                      | 3.5–4.5 mCi                    |
| Collimator   | High resolution                | Low energy, medium resolution  |
| Zoom         | No zoom 10 in. FOV or 1.2–1.5 zoom LFOV | No zoom 10 in. FOV or 1.2–1.5 zoom LFOV |
| Matrix       | 128 × 128                      | 128 × 128                      |
| Peak         | 140 keV 20% centered           | 78 keV 30% centered            |
| Gating       | 8 or 16 frames/cardiac cycle   | 8 frames/cardiac cycle         |
| Imaging time | 5 min (10 min ECG-gated)       | 8–10 (10 min ECG-gated)        |
| Imaging counts | At least $10^6$              | At least 600,000–800,000       |

| *Positioning* | | |
|---|---|---|
| *View* | *Detector Position* | *Patient Position* |
| LAO | Best septal | Supine |
| Anterior | Best septal minus 45° | Supine |
| Left lateral | 0° | Right decubitus |

Key factors to ensure optimal quality planar myocardial perfusion imaging are:

1. Adhere to the acquisition parameters listed in Table 7-1.
2. Bring the camera head as close to the patient's chest as possible.
3. Acquire adequate counts.
4. Reproduce exactly stress and rest patient positioning.

## *Soft Tissue Attenuation in Planar Imaging*

### BREAST (FIG. 7-1)

Soft tissue attenuation, in particular by breasts, is an important problem with planar imaging. In order to recognize breast attenuation, one can acquire in addition to the conventional three-view planar image, low-count images—without moving the patient—with a line source in the FOV that outlines the outer contour of the breast.

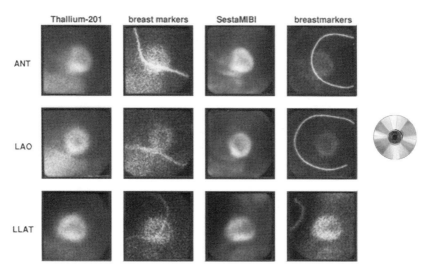

**Fig. 7-1.** Breast markers (i.e., radioactive line sources) applied to planar Tl-201 (thallium-201) and Tc-99m Sestamibi images. The breast markers are taped to a patient's chest and should indicate the outer contour of the breast. If an anterior defect (e.g., on the anterior view of the Tl-201 image) matches the position of the breast marker, the defect is very likely due to breast attenuation.

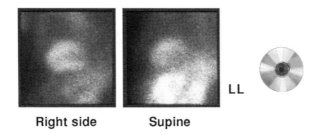

**Fig. 7-2.** Diaphragmatic attenuation is demonstrated in this patient by acquiring two planar left lateral (LL) images in supine and right-side decubitus position. The supine LL image (right) shows an apparent inferobasal perfusion defect. This defect is not present on a second LL image (left) taken a few minutes later with the patient in right side decubitus position. The latter image is normal. Therefore, in the supine position, inferior attenuation is present.

### DIAPHRAGM

Soft tissue attenuation by the left diaphragm is also an important problem with planar images. However, this problem can be entirely avoided by acquiring left lateral images with the patient in a right side decubitus position. (See Fig. 7-2.)

**Table 7-2**
**Processing Steps for Quantification**

| | |
|---|---|
| Background subtraction | Region of interest (ROI), 4 pixels from heart, interpolative background algorithm applied. |
| Image alignment | Slight rotation of images to ensure stress and rest segments correspond accurately. |
| Normalizing images | Scaling of images so the heart is visualized optimally. |
| Quantification | Plot of image count density. |
| Normal database | Allows extent and severity of defect to be calculated. |
| Archiving | Raw and processed data. |

## PROCESSING STEPS FOR QUANTIFICATION

Table 7-2 lists the processing steps for quantification. The following subsections contain comments on the individual items.

### *Background Subtraction*

On planar myocardial projection images there is substantial foreground and background activity projected over the images of the heart. Quantification of regional myocardial uptake cannot be performed without removal of the extracardiac activity. For this purpose "interpolative background correction" was developed *(3)*. A background image is created on the basis of sampling in multiple areas immediately adjacent to the heart and interpolating this information into a new background image. This background image is subsequently subtracted from the raw projection images. The final result of interpolative background correction is a planar image without substantial background that allows for quantitative comparison with normal image files and radiotracer washout. (See Figs. 7-3 and 7-4.)

### *Image Alignment*

For paired quantification of images, it may be necessary to rotate the rest or redistribution image slightly in order to match appropriately with the stress image. Rotation should generally not exceed 20°. (See Fig. 7-5.)

### *Normalizing Images*

Rescaling of the images may be necessary when noncardiac activity is more intense than in the left ventricle. (See Fig. 7-6.)

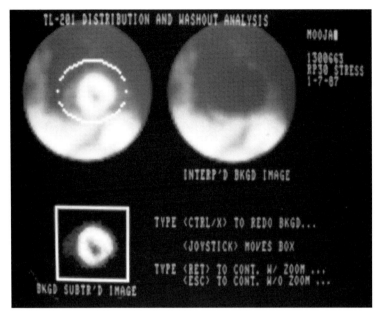

**Fig. 7-3.** Computer screen capture of the process of interpolative background subtraction. The top left image shows an elliptical region of interest placed around the heart for sampling of background counts. The top right image shows the background image created, which is to be subtracted from the original image. The bottom image shows the resulting background-subtracted image of the heart.

## Normal Database

A normal database is generated from images of normal subjects with low (<3%) likelihood of coronary artery disease, based on age, gender, absence of symptoms and risk factors, and normal exercise ECG. From the relative count distribution on images of these normal subjects, a lower limit of normal count distribution, i.e., mean minus two standard deviations, can be derived.

## Quantification

After interpolative background subtraction regional distribution of radiotracer uptake is quantified relative to the myocardial area with maximal uptake. For this purpose the circumference of the left ventricle is divided into a number of segments. The average counts in each segment (from center to periphery) may be displayed as circumferential or transverse profiles that are normalized to local maximal counts. The

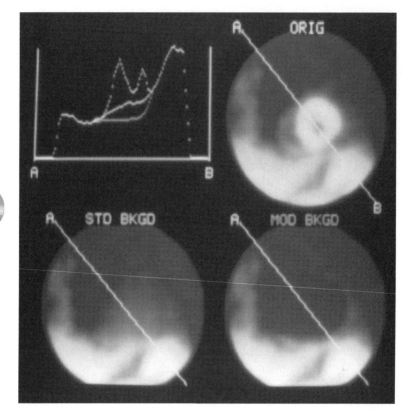

**Fig. 7-4.** Creation of interpolated background images. The top right image shows the original LAO Tc-99m Sestamibi planar myocardial perfusion image. The top left graph shows count profiles through the images from A to B: white = count profile of the original image. The bottom images show the background images created by interpolative substraction. Bottom left: result of standard interpolative background (STD BKGD) as used for Tl-201 (yellow curve in graph) Bottom right: result of modified interpolative background (MOD BKGD) as developed for Tc-99m agents (orange curve in graph). Standard interpolative background subtraction consists of gradually increasing subtraction from low extracardiac counts (lung) to high extracardiac counts (gastrointestinal), thereby leaving a substantial amount of background in the cardiac region. The modified interpolative background substraction initially subtracts a smaller amount of counts from the cardiac region, increasing when the high extracardiac count area is immediately adjacent *(4)*.

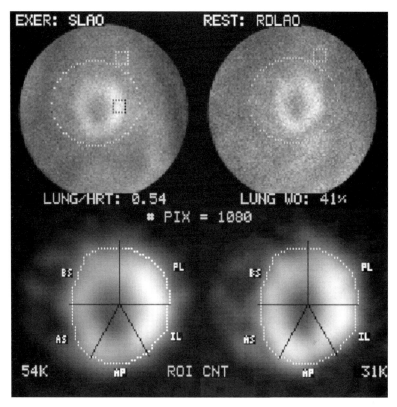

**Fig. 7-5.** First steps in quantification of planar Tl-201 images. Top images: "raw" left anterior oblique (LAO) planar exercise (EXER) and delayed (REST) Tl-201 images. An elliptical region of interest (ROI) is placed around the heart for interpolative background subtraction. The small square ROIs are for calculation of lung/heart (HRT) ratio and lung washout (WO). Bottom images: interpolative background subtracted images of the heart. The exercise and rest images are aligned and five segments are superimposed on the images.

patient's count distribution profiles can be displayed with a lower limit of normal profile. Defect size can then be calculated relative to the normal data files.

## Archiving

All raw image data should be archived daily. It is also useful to archive processed and quantified data for ready comparison with future studies.

## NORMALIZATION TC-99M SESTAMIBI IMAGE

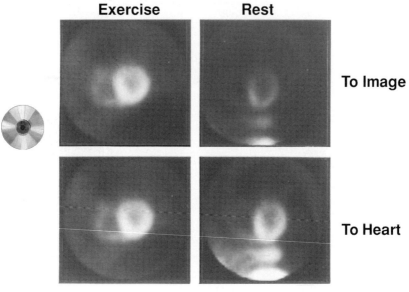

**Fig. 7-6.** Normalization of exercise and rest Tc-99m Sestamibi images. Top: images are normalized to highest counts anywhere within the images. In the exercise image maximal counts are located within the left ventricle. Consequently, the heart is visualized using the full range of the gray scale. In the rest image maximal counts are located outside the left ventricle in the gastrointestinal organs at the bottom of the image. Consequently, the heart is poorly visualized using only the lower end of the gray scale. Bottom: Both exercise and rest images are normalized to maximal counts within the left ventricle. Exercise and rest images can now be compared and interpreted.

## SELECTED BIBLIOGRAPHY

1. DePuey GE, Garcia EV (2001). Updated imaging guidelines for nuclear cardiology procedures, part I. *J Nucl Cardiol* 8:G1–58.
2. ACC/AHA Task force (1995). Guidelines for clinical use of cardiac radionuclide imaging. *J Am Coll Cardiol* 25:521–547.
3. Watson DD, Campbell NP, Read EK, Gibson RS, Teates CD, Beller GA (1981). Spatial and temporal quantitation of plane thallium myocardial images. *J Nucl Med* 22:577–584.
4. Koster K, Wackers FJTh, Mattera J, Fetterman R (1990). Quantitative analysis of planar Tc-99m-Sestamibi myocardial perfusion images using modified background subtraction. *J Nucl Med* 31:1400–1408.

# 8

## Planar Equilibrium Radionuclide Angiocardiography Acquisition and Processing Protocols

> Planar equilibrium radionuclide angiocardiography (ERNA), also known as radionuclide ventriculography (RVG), gated blood pool imaging (GBPI), or MUGA (multigated acquisition), is performed in most laboratories considerably less frequently than radionuclide myocardial perfusion imaging. ERNA is the most reproducible, accurate, and simple method for noninvasively assessing left ventricular ejection fraction (LVEF) *(1,2)*.

ERNAs are now most often used for serial assessment of LVEF in patients who undergo chemotherapy, assessment of global regional wall motion in patients with recent or old myocardial infarction, and in patients with congestive heart failure.

Right ventricular function can be evaluated only by visual inspection on ERNA. Because of overlap by other cardiac structures, RVEF cannot be calculated reliably. The ECG-gated first pass method is an alternative means of calculating RVEF *(3)*.

All acquisition parameters listed in the following tables are based on the Updated imaging guidelines for nuclear cardiology procedures *(4)* (on line: www.asnc.org; menu: library and resources: guidelines and standards). Additional information about accepted standards for performing ERNAs can be found in the Society of Nuclear Medicine Procedure Guidelines for Gated Equilibrium Radionuclide Ventriculography (on line: www.snm.org/policy/new_guidelines_1.html).

**Clinical indications** for nuclear cardiology imaging can be found on line: www.acc.org/clinical/radio/57252.pdf in Guidelines for clinical use of cardiac radionuclide imaging *(5)*.

From: *Contemporary Cardiology: Nuclear Cardiology, The Basics*
F. J. Th. Wackers, W. Bruni, and B. L. Zaret © Humana Press Inc., Totowa, NJ

# ACQUISITION

At the present time most ERNAs are acquired by multiple-view planar imaging technique. Recently, there has been increased interest in acquiring ERNAs by SPECT technology (see chapter 9). The acquisition parameters are given in Table 8-1. The following subsections discuss the individual acquisition parameters. Positions during acquisition are in Table 8-2.

## *Dose and Labeling*

Red blood cells can be labeled using three techniques:

1. In vivo
2. Modified in vivo
3. In vitro

For each of these methods, stannous ion (in the form of stannous pyrophosphate) is used as a reducing agent to facilitate the binding of pertechnetate to hemoglobin.

### In Vivo Labeling

(The labeling efficiency for this method is 60–70%.)

- Inject 10–20 μg/kg of cold stannous pyrophosphate IV.
- After 15–30 min, inject 20–30 mCi of Tc-99m pertechnetate directly intravenously.

### Modified in Vivo Labeling

(The labeling efficiency for this method approaches 90%.)

- Inject 10–20 μg/kg of cold stannous pyrophosphate IV.
- After 15–30 min draw 3 mL of venous blood into a shielded syringe containing the anticoagulant acid-citrate-dextrose and 20–30 mCi of Tc-99m pertechnetate.
- Incubate at room temperature for at least 10 min.
- Re-inject radiolabeled blood into patient.

### In Vitro Labeling

The labeling efficiency for this method is >97%. Presently commercial kits (e.g., Ultratag®) are available that have simplified this method. Therefore, we believe, this technique is the method of choice.

- Three components are required: a vial with stannous chloride dihydrate, sodium dihydrate, and sodium citrate dihydrate; a syringe I with sodium hypochlorite; and a syringe II with citric acid monohydrate and sodium citrate dihydrate.

**Table 8-1**
**Acquisition Parameters**

|  | Rest | Stress[a] |
|---|---|---|
| Dose | 25–30 mCi | |
| Collimator Parallel hole | LEHR Parallel holeL | LEHS |
| Matrix | 64 × 64 | 64 × 64 |
| Zoom | No zoom 10-in. FOV or 1.5–2.2 zoom LFOV | No zoom 10-in. FOV or 1.5–2.2 zoom LFOV |
| Peak | 140 keV 20% centered | 140 keV 20% centered |
| Frame rate | 16 frames/cycle | 16 frames/cycle |
| R-R window | 10–15% | 20–25% |
| Beat rejection | Buffered beat or on the fly | Buffered beat or on the fly |
| Acquisition mode | Frame mode | Frame mode |
| Acquisition length | > 4 million counts standard FOV | 2–2.5 min/stage |
| Pixel size | < 4 mm/pixel | < 4 mm/pixel |

[a]Acquisition parameters for stress ERNA are shown for completeness. In actual practice, exercise ERNAs are infrequently performed in most laboratories.
LEHR = Low-energy high resolution; LEHS = Low-energy high sensitivity.

**Table 8-2**
**Positioning**

| View | Detector position | Patient position |
|---|---|---|
| 1st pass | 5–10° RAO | Supine |
| LAO | Best RV/LV separation (also known as "best septal") | Supine |
| Anterior | Best RV/LV separation minus 45° | Supine |
| Left lateral | Best RV/LV separation plus 45° | Right decubitus |

- Draw 1–3 mL of venous blood into syringe with heparin or anticoagulant citrate dextrose (ACD).
- Add blood to vial and wait 5 min.
- Add content of syringe I to vial and gently mix and invert.
- Add content of syringe II to vial and gently mix and invert.
- Add dose of Tc-99m pertechnetate to vial (in lead-shield container) and gently mix and invert.
- Wait 20 min.
- Re-inject blood into patient.

## *Collimator*

The low-energy high-resolution (LEHR) collimator is used for a rest ERNA. However, when performing exercise ERNAs, the short acquisition time (2 min) of stress images requires the use of a high-sensitivity collimator in order to ensure adequate count statistics. When performing rest and stress ERNAs, one should use the same collimator for both parts. A low-energy all-purpose (LEAP) collimator can be used to increase the sensitivity while still providing adequate image resolution.

## *Matrix*

Any matrix that produces a 4 mm pixel size can be used. A $64 \times 64$ matrix is standard.

## *ECG Gating*

### CHEST ELECTRODES

For ECG gating the computer should receive a clear R-wave signal. Usually three electrodes are used: right and left subclavicular and one on the lateral lower chest (either right or left). If this conventional electrode placement does not work, move the electrodes around to a position that results in a more distinct R-wave. (Make sure that in patients with abnormal ECG or peaked T waves no double signal is detected.)

### NUMBER OF FRAMES

No less than 16 frames/cardiac cycle should be acquired for accurate assessment of LVEF. Although 24 or more frames/cardiac cycle have better temporal resolution and result in better time-activity curves, the acquisition files are too large for most present day nuclear medicine computers.

### R-R WINDOW

A 10–15% window around the R-R peak is standard and accommodates physiologic heart rate variability. Increasing the window beyond this may cause the EF to be less accurate. Nevertheless, during exercise acquisition the window is expanded to 25% in order to accommodate the quickly changing heart rate. The R-R peak also needs to be adjusted at the beginning of each stage in response to the increasing heart rate.

## *Beat Rejection*

Buffered beat rejection means that each beat is temporarily stored in memory to determine if the beat falls within the acceptable R-R window. If the beat is not within the window, it is rejected without contaminating the acquisition. This is the preferred method of beat rejection. Some systems reject beats "on the fly," which means the beat is determined to be bad and rejected as it is seen, but not before a small portion of it is added to the acquisition.

## Acquisition Mode

Forward or forward/backward framing are standard on most systems. An alternative acquisition method is the list mode. List mode allows all beats to be accepted and then the operator selects the beat length to use. This offers more flexibility in window selection but usually requires extra processing time to convert the list mode to frame mode for LVEF calculation. List mode studies also take up much more disk space than frame mode studies. List mode should be used for ECG-gated first pass studies, which are commonly used for assessment of right ventricular ejection fraction.

---

**Atrial Fibrillation**

Meaningful data can be acquired with ERNA in patients with atrial fibrillation using standard ECG-gated acquisition. The calculated LVEF then represents the average LVEF during the time of acquisition. Owing to the varying R-R interval in atrial fibrillation, there is considerable beat-to-beat variation in LVEF values. List mode acquisition can be used to select beats within a specific range of R-R interval.

---

## ECG-Gated First Pass for RVEF

The injection of the Tc-99m-labeled blood cells is used for this purpose. The gamma camera and computer are set up as for acquisition of ERNA *(3)*. Acquisition is started in the right anterior oblique position and the radiolabeled blood is injected rapidly in an antecubital vein. One can either stop acquisition when the radioactive bolus passes through the pulmonary artery, as can be assessed on the persistance scope, or one can acquire the entire first-pass study in list mode and reformat the data later.

## Acquisition Time

Rest ERNAs are usually acquired for counts, not time. It is of crucial importance to have adequate count statistics to ensure reliable and reproducible assessment of LVEF. Using 25–30 mCi, it takes about 5 min to acquire approx 4 million counts with a small FOV camera equipped with a high-resolution collimator. One must keep in mind that if the spleen is abnormally hot, acquisition time needs to be increased, because most of the counts are emanating from the spleen and not the heart.

For stress ERNAs the acquisition time is shortened. Stress ERNAs are acquired during the last 2 min of each 3 min stage of stress.

**Table 8-3**
**Processing Parameters**

| | |
|---|---|
| Smoothing | Nine-point spatial and temporal. |
| Background subtraction | ROI 5–10 pixels from diastolic ROI. |
| ED and ES ROIs | Manual or automated |
| Volume curve generation | Over ROIs, background subtracted |
| RV/LV ejection fraction calculation | Global or regional |
| LV diastolic function | Peak filling rate and time to peak filling rate |
| LV volumes | End diastolic and end systolic volumes |
| Cine or movie generated | Qualitative assessment of wall motion |
| Archiving | Raw and processed data |

## *Pixel Size*

Pixel size should be kept under 4 mm/pixel. Depending on the size of the FOV of the camera, one may have to use a zoom factor to reduce pixel size to <4 mm. Typically a small FOV of 10 in. does not require any zoom. A large FOV can require a zoom from 1.5 to 2.2 depending on the size of the FOV.

## PROCESSING

Similar to acquisition parameters, processing parameters may vary slightly from vendor to vendor. While the processing steps may be different on each computer system, the overall methodology should be similar. Table 8-3 outlines the options computer systems should provide. These processing parameters are also based on the "Updated imaging guidelines for nuclear cardiology procedures" *(4)* (on line: www.asnc.org; menu: library and resources: guidelines and standards).

Table 8-3 lists the processing parameters. The following subsections are comments on the individual items.

## *Background Subtraction*

Vendors differ with respect to the placement of left ventricular background region of interest (ROI). In some programs the ROI is placed automatically 4 pixels outside the lateral border of the end diastolic ROI; in others, the operator is asked to place the background ROI manually. Regardless of the method, the operator must make sure that the background ROI is not placed over an exceedingly hot area, e.g., spleen or descending aorta. A misplaced background region significantly affects the calculation of left ventricular ejection fraction. When the background is too high, LVEF will be erroneously high; conversely when background is too low, LVEF will be too low. For this reason, it is important to archive data that document the selection of background. Background selection should be checked for reproducibility when comparing LVEF on serial studies.

### LV End-Diastolic and End-Systolic Regions of Interest

Many systems have semi- or fully automatic programs that will draw end-diastolic and end-systolic regions of interest (ROI). All ROI's must be checked for accuracy and redrawn manually as necessary. (See **Fig. 8-1**.)

### LV Volume Curve Generation

The appearance of the left ventricular volume curve must be the first item to be checked as part of routine quality control . The curve (**Fig. 8-2**) should start at end diastole (highest counts), then descend to a well-defined and narrow end systolic trough (lowest counts), then demonstrate a smooth diastolic upslope and finally an "atrial kick" that merges with end diastole. It is acceptable that one last frame contains less counts due to respiratory variation in heart rate. However, if a larger number of frames at the end of the cardiac cycle contain low counts due to arrhythmia during acquisition, the diastolic portion of the volume curve is significantly distorted. The volume curve is then unreliable for calculation of diastolic filling parameters. The LV ejection fraction is calculated as follows:

$$\frac{\text{End Diastolic Counts (bc)} - \text{End Systolic Counts (bc)}}{\text{End Diastolic Counts (bc)}}$$

where bc = background corrected. The lower limit of normal for LVEF derived from planar ERNA is 0.50.

### Peak Filling Rate

If ERNAs are acquired with sufficient temporal resolution (24 frames per RR-cycle) or if Fourier curve fitting is performed to 16-frame ERNAs, diastolic filling parameters can be calculated. The lower limit of normal peak filling rate is 2.5 end diastolic volumes/s.

### Volumes

Left ventricular volumes can be derived from ERNAs using a number of methods. This may involve either the acquisition and counting of a reference blood sample, or measuring pixel size for calibration. The

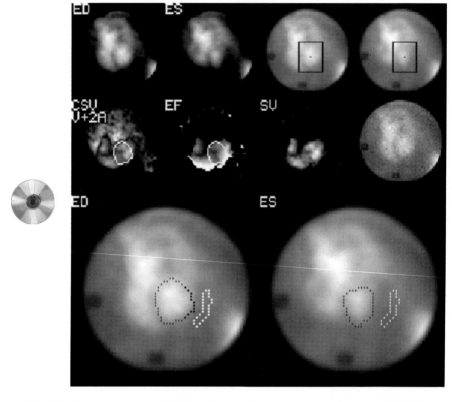

**Fig. 8-1.** Computer screen display of processing parameters of a normal ERNA. On the top right are raw end-diastolic (ED) and end-systolic (ES) frames. The rectangle over the left ventricle is used for automatic search of ED and ES edges. The ED and ES edges are displayed in two larger images on the bottom of the figure for quality control. The automatically placed background region (white dots) is also shown. The images in the middle row left are functional images that may be helpful for assessing whether the edges were assigned correctly.

upper limit of normal end diastolic left ventricular volume is generally between 100 and 140 mL. Discussion of the details of determining volumes is beyond the scope of this book and can be found in the literature *(4)*.

### RV Ejection Fraction

For determination of RV ejection fraction the RV gated first pass data are displayed. A large initial ROI is drawn over the RV and a time-activity curve is plotted to identifying the end systolic frame. Separate ROIs are drawn outlining the end-diastolic and end-systolic contours (**Fig. 8-3**).

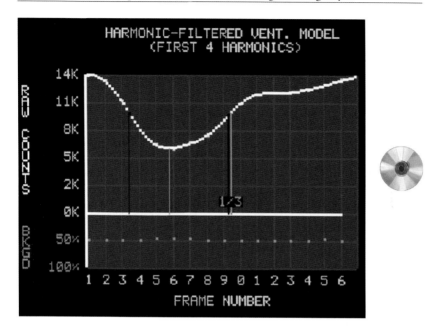

**Fig. 8-2.** Computer screen capture of normal left ventricular volume curve. The curve should be inspected to ensure it displays an appropriate "physiologic" shape.

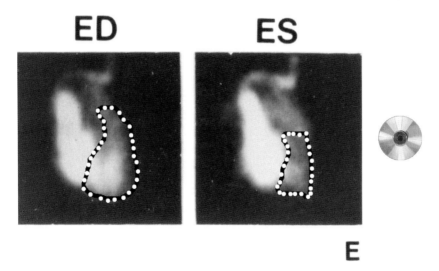

**Fig. 8-3.** Manually drawn regions of interest outlining the end-diastolic (ED) and end-systolic (ES) borders of a normal right ventricle. One should be careful to include the right ventricular outflow tract in the regions of interest.

RVEF is calculated in the usual manner. No background subtraction is necessary. Note: count density may be suboptimal in about 10% of patients. If counts in the end diastolic ROI are less than 1000, RVEF should not be calculated. The lower limit of normal RVEF is 0.42 *(3)*.

## *Archiving*

All raw data should be archived daily. Storing documentation of processing and quantified data for comparison with future studies is recommended.

## SELECTED BIBLIOGRAPHY

1. Wackers FJTh, Berger HJ, Johnstone DE, et al. (1979). Multiple gated cardiac blood pool imaging for left ventricular ejection fraction: validation of the technique and assessment of variability. *Am J Cardiol* 43:1159–1166.
2. van Royen N, Jaffe CC, Krumholz HK, et al. (1996). Comparison and reproducibility of visual echocardiographic and quantitative radionuclide left ventricular ejection fraction. *Am J Cardiol* 77:843–850.
3. Winzelberg GG, Boucher CA, Pohost GM, et al. (1981). Right ventricular function in aortic and mitral valve disease: relation of gated first pass radionuclide angiography to clinical and hemodynamic findings. *Chest* 79:520–528.
4. DePuey GE, Garcia EV (2001). Updated imaging guidelines for nuclear cardiology procedures, part I. *J Nucl Cardiol* 8:G1–58.
5. ACC/AHA Task force (1995). Guidelines for clinical use of cardiac radionuclide imaging. *J Am Coll Cardiol* 25:521–547.
6. Levy WC, Cerqueira MD, Matsuoka DT, Harp GD, Sheehan FH, Stratton JR. (1992). Four radionuclide methods for left ventricular volume determinations: comparison of a manual and automated technique. *J Nucl Med* 33:763–770.

# 9

# SPECT Equilibrium Radionuclide Angiocardiography Acquisition and Processing Protocols

SPECT ERNA is not routinely performed in most nuclear cardiology laboratories. Although the equipment used for the acquisition of ECG-gated SPECT myocardial perfusion images allows for acquisition of ECG-gated SPECT ERNA without additional hardware or modifications, the processing software and the calculation of global LVEF is not fully standardized and/or widely validated. It is likely that in the near future SPECT ERNA will be utilized with increasing frequency.

The greatest attraction of SPECT ERNA is in the ability to evaluate cardiac chambers and regional wall motion without overlap of other structures.

LVEF may be calculated based on count changes from either a conventional planar LAO image or from SPECT LVEF long-axis slices. SPECT ERNA LVEF generally is higher than planar ERNA LVEF.

All acquisition parameters listed in the following tables are based on the "Updated imaging guidelines for nuclear cardiology procedures, Part 1" *(1)* (on line: www.asnc.org; menu: library and resources: guidelines and standards).

**Clinical indications** for nuclear cardiology imaging can be found on line: www.acc.org/clinical/radio/57252.pdf Guidelines for clinical use of cardiac radionuclide imaging *(2)*. (These guidelines are currently being revised.)

From: *Contemporary Cardiology: Nuclear Cardiology, The Basics*
F. J. Th. Wackers, W. Bruni, and B. L. Zaret © Humana Press Inc., Totowa, NJ

**Table 9-1**
**Acquisition Parameters**

|  |  | Rest |
|---|---|---|
| Dose |  | 30 mCi |
| Collimator |  | LEHR Parallel hole |
| Matrix |  | 64 × 64 |
| Zoom |  | No zoom 10-in. FOV or 1.5–2.2 zoom LFOV |
| Peak |  | 140 keV 20% centered |
| Frame rate |  | 16 frames/cycle |
| R-R window | 25–35% |  |
| Beat rejection |  | On the fly |
| Acquisition mode | Frame mode |  |
| Number of stops |  | 64 |
| Time/stop |  | 30 s |
| Pixel size |  | 4–5 mm |
| Planar LAO | 5 min acquisition (for calculation of LVEF) | |

## ACQUISITION PARAMETERS

Table 9-1 lists the acquisition parameters. The following subsections comment on the individual parameters.

### Collimator

Because of abundance of counts, a parallel hole LEHR collimator is preferred.

### Pixel Size

Usually a 64 × 64 matrix with the appropriate zoom will produce a 4–5 mm/pixel. Depending on the size of the FOV of the camera, one may have to adjust the zoom to obtain the correct pixel size. Typically a small FOV of 10 in. does not require any zoom. A large FOV can require a zoom from 1.5 to 1.75 depending on the exact size of the FOV.

### ECG Gating

#### CHEST ELECTRODES

For ECG gating the computer should receive a clear R-wave signal. Usually three electrodes are used: right and left subclavicular and one on the lateral lower chest (either right or left). If this conventional electrode placement does not work, move the electrodes around to a position that results in a more distinct R-wave. (Make sure that in patients with abnormal ECG or peaked T waves no double signal is detected.)

### Number of Frames

Sixteen frames per cardiac cycle are preferred over 8 frames/cycle. As is the case for SPECT myocardial perfusion-derived LVEF (see p. 64), calculation from data acquired with 8 frames/cycle may decrease value of LVEF *(3)*.

### R-R Window

The window width is larger for SPECT ERNA than for planar ERNA in order to increase the count statistics. A 25–35% window is standard; however, it may vary with different camera systems and with the underlying cardiac rhythm.

## Beat Rejection

This parameter may also differ from system to system. An "on the fly" beat rejection where the abnormal beat and the subsequent beat are rejected is preferred.

## Acquisition Mode

Frame mode is standard on most systems.

## Number of Projections

Thirty-two projections per head over 180° are adequate. For dual-headed systems with the camera heads at 90°, a total of 64 stops would be acquired.

## Time per Stop

Total acquisition time is approx 20 min. For a dual-headed system acquiring 64 projections, each stop would be 30 s.

## PROCESSING PARAMETERS

Table 9-2 lists the processing parameters. The following subsections comment on the individual parameters.

## Filtering

The purpose of image filters is to remove noise and blur before and after back projection of raw SPECT data. The standard filter for SPECT imaging is the Butterworth filter. The optimal order and cutoff of this filter are different for each vendor.

## Motion Correction

Not all programs are capable of correcting ECG-gated data. Check with the vendor. After applying the program to the data always check the

### Table 9-2
### Processing Parameters

| | |
|---|---|
| Filtering | Filtered back projection is standard, cutoffs and frequencies are vendor dependent. |
| Motion correction | Some programs are not able to correct gated data. |
| Reconstruction | Reorienting of data into vertical and horizontal long axis and short axis planes. |
| Normalizing cine | The gray scale setting normalized to heart activity. |
| Ejection fraction | Derived from count changes within ventricular region of interest. |
| Volumes | Simpson's rule: sum of pixels within each slice, summed for all slices. |
| Archiving | Raw and processed data. |

reconstructed slices for motion artifacts. The programs are not fool proof and are not always successful.

## Reconstruction

This step reorients the data to the three axes of the patient's heart. Horizontal long-axis, vertical long-axis, and short-axis slices are created.

## Normalizing Slices

This step may be necessary if the patient has intense radiotracer uptake in the spleen. When images are normalized to the spleen, the heart may not be visible. The gray scale setting must be normalized to the maximal pixel value within the heart for optimal visualization of cardiac structures.

## Left Ventricular Volume Curve Generation

A volume curve can be generated using either hand-drawn or automatically generated multiple ROIs over the summed short axis slices including the entire left ventricle and excluding the left atrium. Automatically generated ROIs should be checked for accuracy.

## Left Ventricular Ejection Fraction

Not many well-validated software packages exist to determine SPECT ERNA LVEF. LVEF can be determined from the change in counts in the summed short-axis end-diastolic and summed short-axis end-systolic ROIs using the following conventional formula:

$$\frac{\text{End diastolic counts} - \text{End systolic counts}}{\text{End diastolic counts}}$$

Because left ventricular background in reconstructed SPECT images is extremely low, no background subtraction is necessary.

LVEF by SPECT ERNA is found to be higher (1.4× planar LVEF-8) than by planar ERNA because lack of atrial overlap *(4,5)*. The lower limit of normal SPECT LVEF is about 0.60.

## *Left Ventricular Volumes*

Right and left ventricular volumes have been determined from SPECT ERNA using a modified Simpson's rule and found to correlate well with volumes derived from magnetic resonance imaging *(6)*.

## *Archiving*

All raw data should be archived daily. It is also recommended that processed and quantified data be stored for comparison with future studies.

## SELECTED BIBLIOGRAPHY

1. DePuey GE, Garcia EV (2001). Updated imaging guidelines for nuclear cardiology procedures, part I. *J Nucl Cardiol* 8:G1–58.
2. ACC/AHA Task Force (1995). Guidelines for clinical use of cardiac radionuclide imaging. *J Am Coll Cardiol* 25:521–547.
3. Germano G, Kiat H, Kavanagh PB, et al. (1995). Automatic quantification of ejection fraction from gated myocardial perfusion SPECT. *J Nucl Med* 36:2138–2147.
4. Bartlett ML, Srinivasan G, Barker WC, Kitsiou AN, Dilsizian V, Bacharach SL (1996). Left ventricular ejection fraction: comparison of results from planar and SPECT gated blood-pool studies. *J Nucl Med* 37:1795–1799.
5. Groch MW, DePuey EG, Belzberg AC, et al. (2001). Planar imaging versus gated blood-pool SPECT for assessment of ventricular performance: a multicenter study. *J Nucl Med* 42:1773–1779.
6. Chin BB, Bloomgarden DC, Xia W, et al. (1997). Right and left ventricular volume and ejection fraction by tomographic gated blood-pool scintigraphy. *J Nucl Med* 38:942–948.

# 10 Display and Analysis of SPECT Myocardial Perfusion Images

The display and nomenclature of nuclear cardiology images have been standardized. The analysis of nuclear cardiology images should follow a systematic approach and sequence as outlined in the Imaging Guidelines for Nuclear Cardiology Procedures, Part 2 *(1)* (on line: www.asnc.org; menu: library and resources: guidelines and standards).

## DISPLAY OF SPECT MYOCARDIAL PERFUSION IMAGES

**The display of SPECT myocardial perfusion images should include at a minimum:**

- Rotating planar projection images
- Reconstructed slices
- Movie display of selected ECG-gated slices
- Three-dimensional condensation of image data

**The interpretation of SPECT myocardial perfusion images should follow a systematic approach:**

1. Inspection of rotating planar projection images (**Fig. 10-1**).
2. Analysis of reconstructed tomographic short axis, vertical and long axis slices.
3. Analysis of regional and global left ventricular function.
4. Incorporation of quantitative perfusion and functional data.
5. Incorporation of clinical and stress data.
6. Final interpretation and report.

The individual planar projection images should be viewed on computer screen in a rotating endless loop cine format.

**The rotating images should be inspected for**

1. Overall quality of images
2. Motion and effectiveness of motion correction

From: *Contemporary Cardiology: Nuclear Cardiology, The Basics*
F. J. Th. Wackers, W. Bruni, and B. L. Zaret © Humana Press Inc., Totowa, NJ

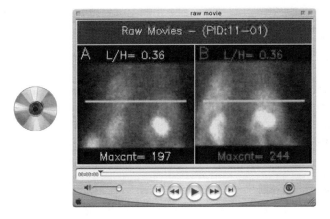

**Fig. 10-1.** Rotating planar projection images of a SPECT study. The stress images are on the left, the rest images are on the right. The maximal counts per pixel (Maxcnt) within the heart are displayed. The lung-to-heart count ratio (L/H) is also displayed.

3. Gastrointestinal uptake
4. Breast attenuation
5. Diaphragmatic attenuation
6. Count density within the heart
7. Presence of noncardiac radiotracer uptake:
   Lungs
   Thyroid gland
   Salivary glands
   Kidneys
   Tumors and lymph nodes

The overall quality of SPECT images is determined by a number of interrelated variables, such as presence of patient motion and adequacy of motion correction, the intensity and location of gastrointestinal uptake, breast or diaphragmatic attenuation, and, very importantly, count density in the heart.

**EVALUATION OF ROTATION PLANAR PROJECTION IMAGES**

**Count density and image inspection**
There are several ways to assess count density, e.g., total counts in the entire SPECT study or per planar projection image. We found empirically that the maximal counts per pixel within the left ventricle is a useful measure of quality. When maximal counts in the heart are

< 100 / pixel, reconstructed slices are frequently noisy and of subop-timal quality. Count density can be enhanced either by administering a higher dose of radiopharmaceutical or by prolonging acquisition time. However, in obese patients, even if measured counts are adequate, scattered photons may substantially degrade image quality.

**Patient motion**

Patient motion can **best** be recognized on the rotating planar pro-jection images. This is done by visual inspection. A horizontal line that is aligned with the left ventricular apex is very helpful (see also Chapter 14, p. 149).

**Gastrointestinal uptake**

Images acquired with Tc-99m-labeled agents, in particular those acquired at rest and after pharmacological stress, at times display substantial subdiaphragmatic gastrointestinal uptake. The most dis-turbing image pattern is that of a bowel loop with intense radiotracer uptake immediately adjacent to the left ventricular inferior wall. This may obscure visualization of the inferior wall. The intense uptake may also create artifactual inferior defects due to errors in filtered back projection. On the other hand, fixed inferior defects may appear reversible due to scattered photons from adjacent intense noncardiac uptake. No good remedies exist to avoid these problems. In our expe-rience the best solution is either to wait and repeat imaging later, or to have the patient drink large amounts of fluid in order to move radioactivity further down the gastrointestinal tract.

**Breast shadow**

When viewing the cine display of the rotating planar projection images, one may see the shadow of the left breast moving over the heart from the left anterior oblique to left lateral projections. On pla-nar images breast attenuation is a serious problem that may make images uninterpretable. However, on SPECT imaging, because of the limited number of projections affected, breast attenuation artifacts are not a serious problem most of the time.

**Inferior attenuation**

On cine display of the rotating planar projection images, one may see a sudden disappearance of the inferior wall in the left lateral projections. Such a sudden disappearance favors diaphragmatic attenuation, whereas a gradual appearance of an inferior wall defect makes it more likely that a true myocardial perfusion defect is present.

**ECG-gating problems**

ECG-gating problems may be suspected by reviewing the cine display of the planar projection images. Sometimes a "flashing" effect occurs, caused by brighter and darker projection images. If the heart rate during SPECT image acquisition was irregular, not all 8 or 16 bins of an ECG-gated SPECT study have accumulated the same number of counts per stop, resulting in darker and lighter images. However, one should be aware that ECG-gating irregularities are often subtle and may not be spotted directly from planar projection images.

**Localized noncardiac radiotracer uptake**

Depending on the size of the FOV, rotating projection images also display part of the chest and upper abdomen. When inspecting rotating images, one should pay attention to normal and abnormal extracardiac radiotracer accumulation. One may see varying degrees of uptake in the salivary glands, thyroid gland and stomach mucosa. This is not abnormal and is due to the presence of free unlabeled Tc-99m pertechnetate. At times the skeleton may be faintly visualized; the significance of the latter is unclear. However, localized radiotracer accumulation in the mediastinum, breast(s), and axilla should be considered abnormal and may indicate malignancy. Such abnormal extracardiac uptake should be mentioned in the final report to the referring physician and further clinical work-up should be suggested.

**Increased lung uptake**

Increased radiotracer lung uptake, in particular when present on stress images and not on rest images, is a sign of transient left ventricular dysfunction during stress. Lung uptake is quantified as lung/heart ratio. The lower limit of normal lung/heart ratio is 0.50 for Tl-201 and 0.42 for Tc-99m-Sestamibi or Tetrofosmin.

## *Reconstructed Slices*

The display of reconstructed SPECT slices has been standardized *(1–3)* (**Fig. 10-2**). Three sets of tomographic slices are reconstructed: short axis slices, horizontal long axis slices, and vertical long axis slices. The stress (A) and rest or delayed (B) images are displayed in two rows of images (stress on top and rest below) to facilitate comparison (**Fig. 10-3**). The short-axis images are displayed from apex (left) to base (right). The vertical long-axis slices from septum (left) to lateral wall (right). The horizontal long-axis are displayed from inferior wall (left) to anterior wall (right).

Images are preferably displayed on computer screen in color or "white on black" using a linear gray scale. It is important that the display of images is standardized and not changed randomly. Certain color scales have a tendency to exaggerate subtle differences in myocardial radiotracer uptake, other color scales may have the opposite effect.

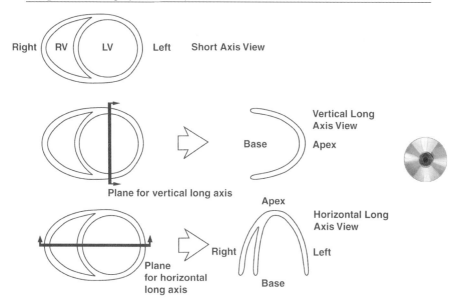

**Fig. 10-2.** Standardized planes of cut for reconstructed SPECT slices. (Reproduced with permission from ref. *2.*)

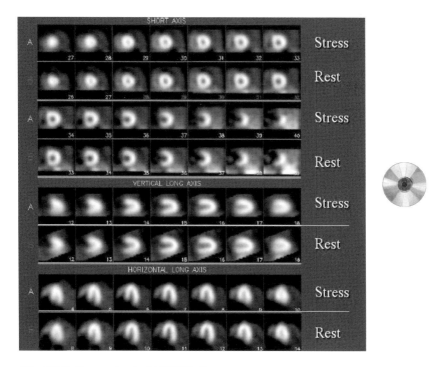

**Fig. 10-3.** Reconstructed SPECT slices.

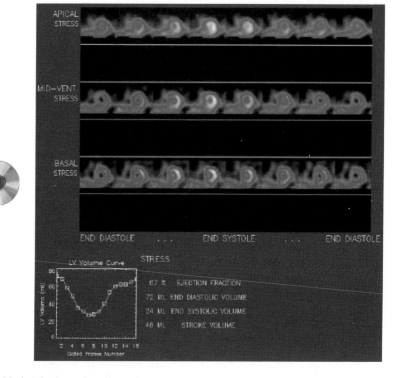

**Fig. 10-4.** Display of wall motion and LVEF of ECG-gated SPECT.

## DISPLAY OF SPECT MYOCARDIAL PERFUSION IMAGES

Reconstructed slices (**Fig. 10-3**) should be checked as to whether tomographic cuts were performed along appropriately selected left ventricular anatomical axes. Inappropriate orientation should be suspected when the morphology of the left ventricle is apparently distorted.

In addition, appropriate alignment of the stress and rest slices should be verified: left ventricular cavity size should be approximately similar on companion stress–rest short-axis slices. Also paired stress–rest long-axis slices should have similar morphology. Obviously when transient ischemic dilation is present, stress and rest images are different and this should be differentiated from misalignment.

ECG-gated SPECT slices are displayed in color and played as an endless loop movie (**Fig. 10-4** and CD Rom). Gradual change in color intensity during the cardiac cycle correlates with left ventricular regional myocardial wall thickening. Problems with ECG-gating should be suspected when the transition from one frame to another shows an abrupt change in intensity ("flashing").

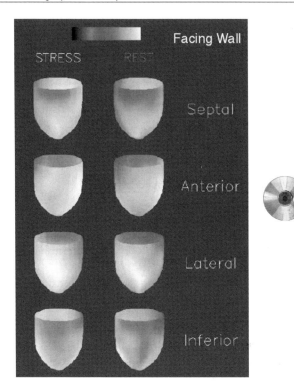

**Fig. 10-5.** Three-dimensional display of myocardial perfusion.

Three-dimensional rendering of myocardial perfusion is shown in **Fig. 10-5**. A composite three-dimensional rendering of myocardial perfusion information from all reconstructed slices is often helpful when myocardial perfusion abnormalities are large. Visualization of the abnormal areas in three dimensions may make it easier to understand the full anatomic involvement of the left ventricle.

## ANALYSIS OF SPECT IMAGES

After quality assurance on display of rotating planar projection images as outlined above, reconstructed slices should first be analyzed visually and then, when available, by quantitative analysis.

Stress and rest reconstructed slices are often divided in 17 segments according to standards developed by the AHA, ACC, and ASNC *(3)*. Specific segments can be assigned to various coronary artery perfusion territories as shown in **Fig. 10-6**.

Because of the many reconstructed SPECT images available for analysis, it is useful to compress all information into *one* image. This can be

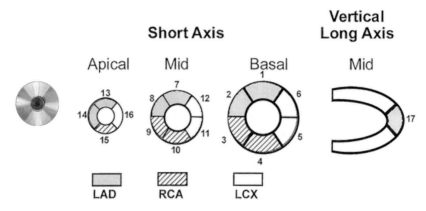

**Fig. 10-6.** Assignment of myocardial segments to the territories of the left anterior descending (LAD), right coronary artery (RCA), and the left circumflex coronary artery (LCX). (Reproduced with permission from ref. *1*.)

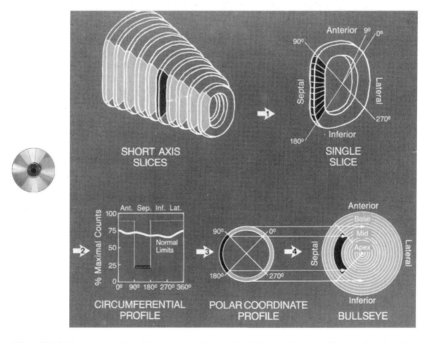

**Fig. 10-7.** Steps involved in generating a "bull's eye" map. (Reproduction by permission of General Electric, Milwaukee, WI.)

done by either displaying a three-dimensional rendering of myocardial perfusion of the left ventricle (**Fig. 10-5**), or by generating color-coded polar maps or "bull's-eye" images (**Fig. 10-7**).

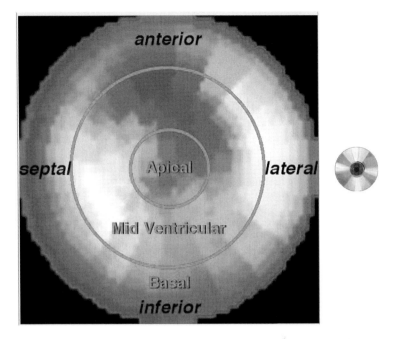

**Fig. 10-8.** Bull's eye display of tomographic myocardial perfusion images.

A bull's eye display of tomographic myocardial perfusion images is shown in **Fig. 10-8**. Myocardial perfusion image data are projected onto one plane. Image data of the apex are projected in the center of the bull's eye. Image data of the base of the left ventricle are projected on the periphery of the bull's eye, whereas mid ventricular image data are projected between these two areas. The location of the anterior, lateral, inferior, and septal walls are indicated. A standardized segmentation and nomenclature for bull's eye display or circumferential polar plot of tomographic myocardial perfusion images *(2,3)* is shown in **Fig. 10-9**. **Figure 10-10** shows a bull's eye display and assignment of coronary artery territories (LAD = left anterior descending coronary artery; LCX = left circumflex coronary artery; RCA = right coronary artery).

## SEMIQUANTITATIVE ANALYSIS

Myocardial perfusion images should not be interpreted simply in a binary fashion as either "normal" or "abnormal," but should be characterized by the degree of decreased radiotracer uptake. Table 10-1 shows a visual semiquantitative scoring method that has been widely used.

By applying the scoring system for each segment of the 17-segment model to both rest and stress images, a summed stress score (SSS), a

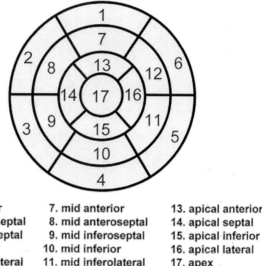

1. basal anterior          7. mid anterior          13. apical anterior
2. basal anteroseptal      8. mid anteroseptal       14. apical septal
3. basal inferoseptal      9. mid inferoseptal       15. apical inferior
4. basal inferior         10. mid inferior          16. apical lateral
5. basal inferolateral    11. mid inferolateral     17. apex
6. basal anterolateral    12. mid anterolateral

**Fig. 10-9.** Left ventricular segmentation. (Reproduced with permission from ref. *1*.)

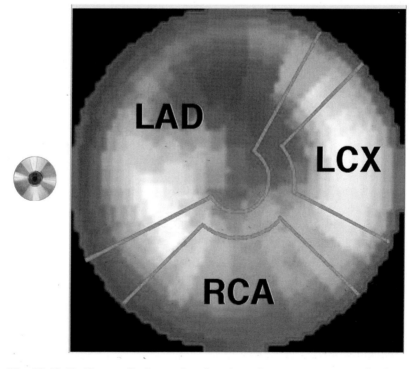

**Fig. 10-10.** Bull's eye display and assignment of coronary artery territories.

**Table 10-1**
**Semiquantitative Scoring**

| | |
|---|---|
| Normal = | 0 |
| Mildly reduced = | 1 |
| Moderately reduced = | 2 |
| Severely reduced = | 3 |
| Absent uptake = | 4 |

summed rest score (SRS), and a summed difference score (SDS) can be derived. These semiquantitative scores have been shown to provide important prognostic information. A normal image thus has a score of "0," whereas the maximal abnormal score is "68" (no heart visualized). A summed score of <8 is considered small, 9–13 moderate, and >13 large.

## QUANTITATIVE ANALYSIS

Radionuclide imaging is an intrinsically digital technique that is ideally suited for quantification. A number of validated software packages are commercially available for quantification of SPECT myocardial perfusion and function (QPS-QGS™; Emory Toolbox™; 4D-MSPECT™; and Wackers-Liu CQ™), and are carried by the major vendors of nuclear medicine imaging equipment *(4–7)*.

The basic principles of SPECT quantification are similar for each of these software packages. Normalized relative radiotracer uptake in reconstructed slices is quantitatively compared to normal data files. Relative radiotracer uptake on SPECT images is displayed either as polar or bull's eye plots, as was shown above, or as circumferential count distribution profiles. The size of myocardial perfusion defects can be expressed either as percentage of left ventricle, or computer-generated summed stress scores.

Each commercially available package also includes software for computation of LVEF and left ventricular volumes from ECG-gated SPECT images. Ejection fraction calculations are based on applying Simpson's rule to computer-derived endocardial edges and volumes throughout the cardiac cycle.

### *Examples of Commercial Quantitative Software*

**Figures 10-11–10-37** show representative screen captures of the display of four commercially available software packages. Although all examples show anterior wall perfusion abnormalities, the image data are from different patients. (Color versions are on the accompanying CD Rom.)

# CEDARS SINAI QPS AND QGS® (COURTESY GUIDO GERMANO, PhD)

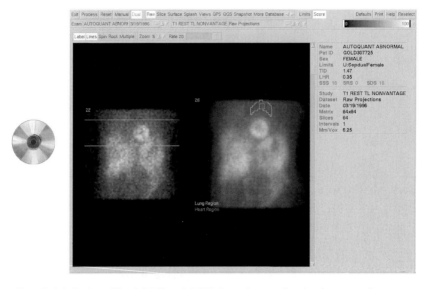

**Fig. 10-11.** Cedars-Sinai QPS and QGS. Rotating projection images of separate acquisition dual-isotope SPECT. Regions of interest for calculating lung/heart ratio are shown.

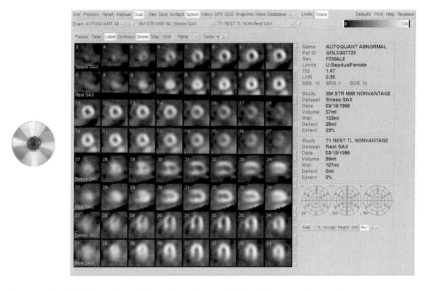

**Fig. 10-12.** Cedars-Sinai QPS and QGS. Standard display of reconstructed tomographic slices. A reversible anteroapical defect is present. On the right quantitative parameters are displayed.

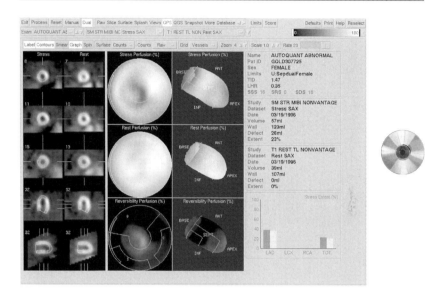

**Fig. 10-13.** Cedars-Sinai QPS and QGS. Quantification of myocardial perfusion. Computer-generated left ventricular contours are displayed on the left. Two-dimensional polar plots (bull's eyes) and three-dimensional rendering of myocardial perfusion are shown in the middle and on the right. On the far right are quantitative results. Summed stress score is 16.

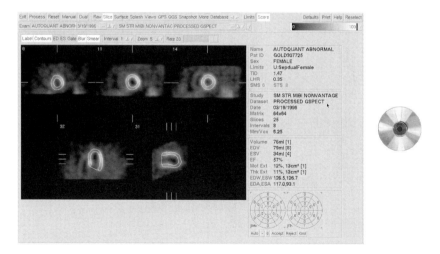

**Fig. 10-14.** Cedars-Sinai QPS and QGS. Left ventricular contours used for calculation of LVEF are displayed. LVEF is 57%.

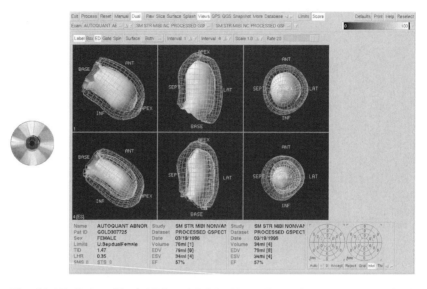

**Fig. 10-15.** Cedars-Sinai QPS and QGS. Three-dimensional rendering of left ventricular function . The end diastolic volume is shown as a bird cage.

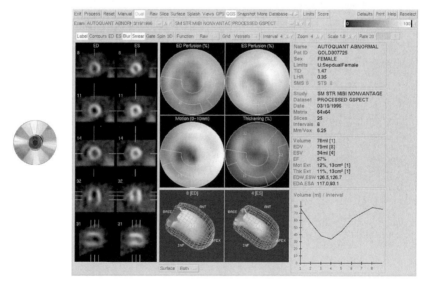

**Fig. 10-16.** Cedars-Sinai QPS and QGS. Summary of quantification of left ventricular perfusion and function. LVEF = 57%.

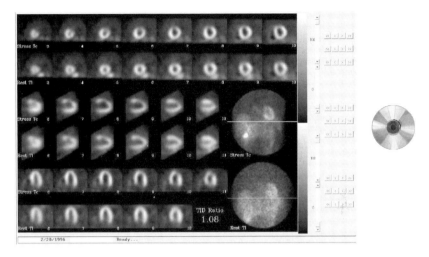

**Fig. 10-17.** Emory Toolbox. Rotating projection images and reconstructed slices of separate acquisition dual-isotope SPECT are displayed. A largely reversible anteroapical myocardial perfusion defect is present

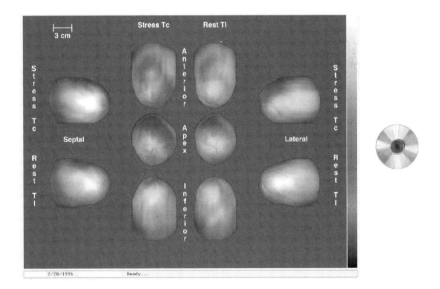

**Fig. 10-18.** Emory Toolbox. Three-dimensional display of myocardial perfusion. The darkened area represents the anteroapical perfusion defect.

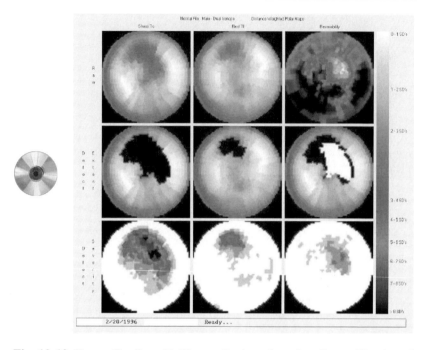

**Fig. 10-19.** Emory Toolbox. Bull's eye display of results of quantification of myocardial perfusion. The anteroapical defect is mostly reversible with small residual rest defect.

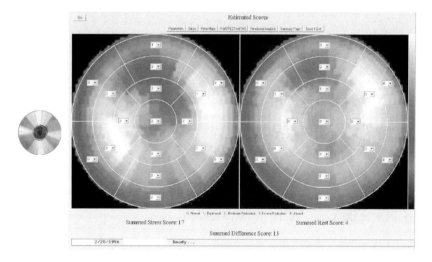

**Fig. 10-20.** Emory Toolbox. Results of quantification. Stress and rest score are computed for each of 17 segments. The summed stress score is 17; summed rest score is 4 and the summed difference score is 13.

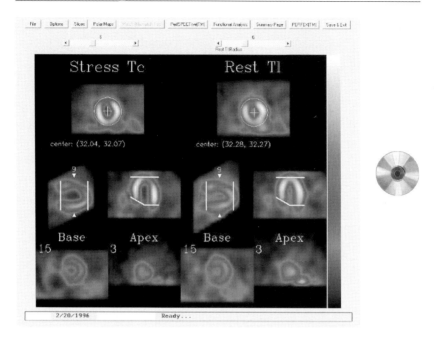

**Fig. 10-21.** Emory Toolbox. Parameters used for computing LVEF from ECG-gated SPECT.

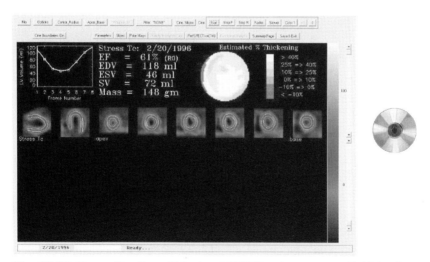

**Fig. 10-22.** Emory Toolbox. Calculated LVEF and percent wall thickening. LVEF is 61% with normal (>40%) wall thickening. End diastole volume is calculated as 118 mL.

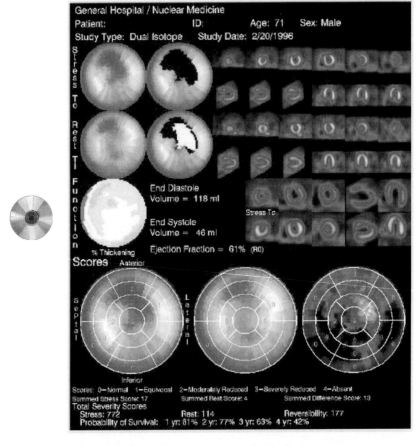

**Fig. 10-23.** Emory Toolbox. Summary screen displaying quantitative myocardial perfusion and function. There is a large, almost completely reversible, anteroseptal myocardial perfusion defect with preserved global and regional left ventricular function.

# 4DM-SPECT® (Courtesy Edward Ficaro, PhD)

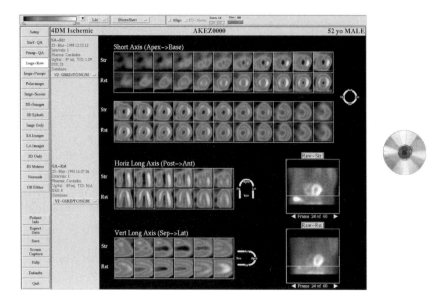

**Fig. 10-24.** 4DM-SPECT. Rotating planar projection images and selected reconstructed slices.

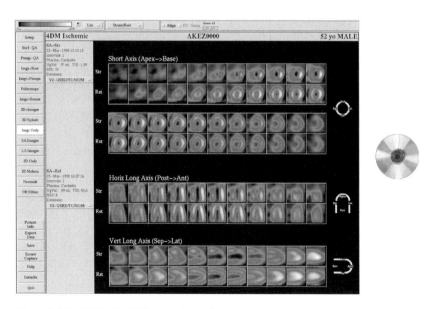

**Fig. 10-25.** 4DM-SPECT. Standard display of reconstructed slices. A reversible anteroapical and septal myocardial perfusion defect is present.

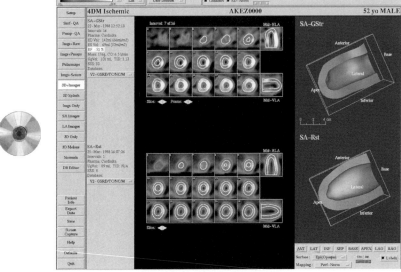

**Fig. 10-26.** 4DM-SPECT. Left ventricular contours for quantifying myocardial perfusion (left) and three-dimensional rendering (right).

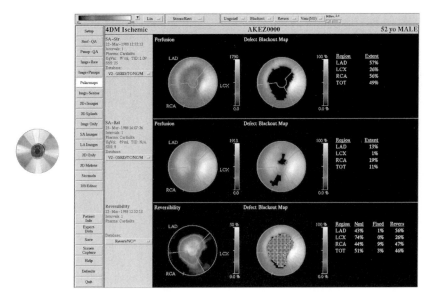

**Fig. 10-27.** 4DM-SPECT. Left column: polar maps of stress (top) and rest (middle) myocardial perfusion and defect reversibility (bottom). Middle column: blackout maps for stress and rest myocardial perfusion in comparison to normal database. Defect sizes in various coronary artery territories are shown on the right.

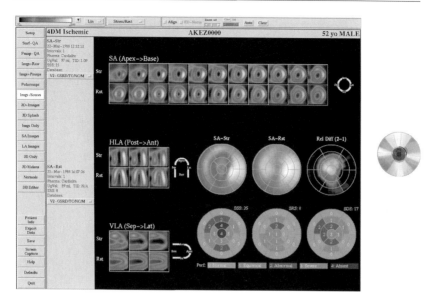

**Fig. 10-28.** 4DM-SPECT. Summary screen of quantitative myocardial perfusion. Summed stress defect size is 25.

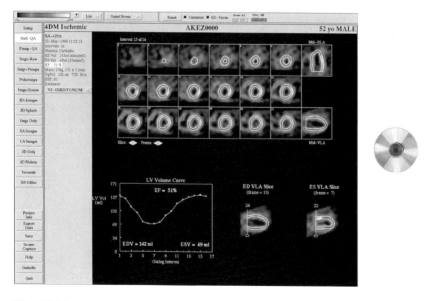

**Fig. 10-29.** 4DM-SPECT. Quantification of left ventricular function. Endocardial and epicardial edges are displayed. Left ventricular volume curve, calculated LVEF and end diastolic and end systolic volumes are shown.

# WACKERS–LIU CARDIAC QUANTIFICATION (WLCQ®)

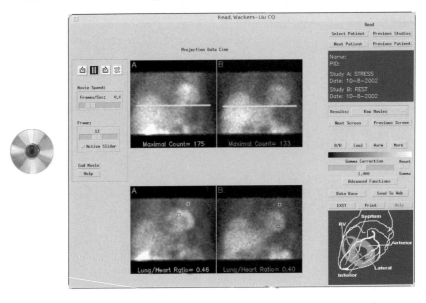

**Fig. 10-30.** WLCQ. Rotating planar projection images and regions of interest for calculating lung/heart ratio.

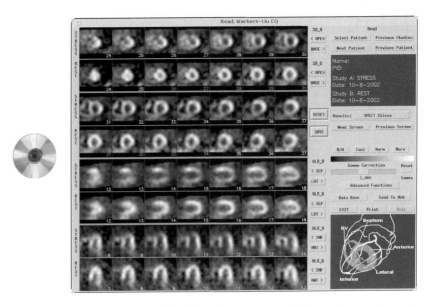

**Fig. 10-31.** WLCQ. Standard display of reconstructed slices of same-day rest-stress Tc-99m-Sestamibi SPECT images. A large reversible anteroseptal and lateral and inferoseptal myocardial perfusion defect is present.

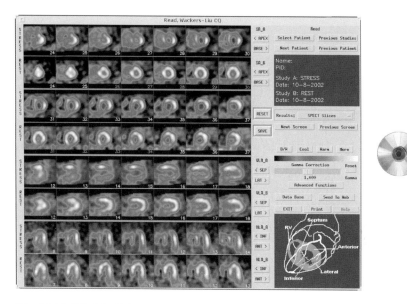

**Fig. 10-32.** WLCQ. Color display of the reconstructed slices displayed in Fig 10-31.

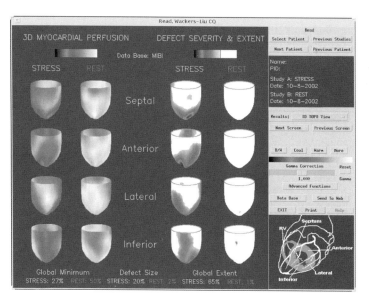

**Fig. 10-33.** WLCQ. Three-dimensional rendering of stress and rest myocardial perfusion. From the top to bottom the septal, anterior, lateral and inferior walls are facing the observer. On the left, regional radiotracer uptake is normalized to maximal count density within the left ventricle. The darkened areas represent decreased myocardial perfusion. On the stress images a large anteroseptal, lateral, and inferior area with decreased uptake can be seen. On the rest images mildly decreased uptake in the inferior wall consistent with attenuation is present. On the right, regional myocardial perfusion is compared to a normal database. Areas with less than normal myocardial uptake are displayed in color. On the stress images a large anteroseptal, lateral, and inferior myocardial perfusion defect can be appreciated. The rest images are normal.

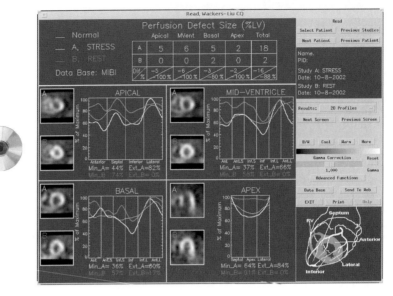

**Fig. 10-34.** WLCQ. Quantification of myocardial perfusion using circumferential count distribution profiles. The yellow curves represent regional count distribution on the stress images. The red curves represent rest images. The white curve depicts the lower limit of normal radiotracer distribution. The stress curve is below the lower limit of normal in the apical slices in the anterior and lateral regions. The rest curve in the apical slices is within normal range. In the mid ventricular short-axis slices, the stress curve is below to the lower limit of normal in the anterior, inferior, and lateral regions. The mid ventricular rest curve is within normal range. In the basal slices the stress curve is below normal in the inferior and lateral region. The rest curve in the basal slices is largely within normal range. At the apex a reversible defect is present. Stress and rest defect size are quantified in the table at the top. The stress defect is large and involves 18% of the left ventricle, the rest defect is very small at 2%. This is an example of a large reversible anteroapical, anteroseptal, lateral and inferior defect.

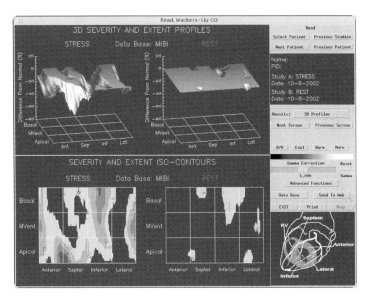

**Fig. 10-35.** WLCQ. Three-dimensional display of circumferential count distribution profiles. The images on top display 36 circumferential count profiles from apex (front) to base (back). The limit of normal myocardial perfusion is displayed as a flat plane. Where the circumferential profile breaks through the normal limits, i.e., abnormal perfusion, valleys are shown. On the stress profiles (left), abnormal perfusion ('valleys") is present in the anterior, septal, and lateral regions. On the rest images (right) only mild impressions are present at the base in the inferolateral walls. The bottom images show color-coded projections of the image on top. Dark-blue is normal. Abnormal perfusion is indicated by shades of color. This rectangular display is similar to the concentric bull's eye display. However, the apical myocardial perfusion data are displayed at the bottom of the rectangle and the basal perfusion data are displayed at the top of the rectangle. This leads to less distortion of the extent of myocardial perfusion abnormalities than with the concentric bull's eye display. The marked reversibility of stress-induced myocardial perfusion abnormality can be appreciated.

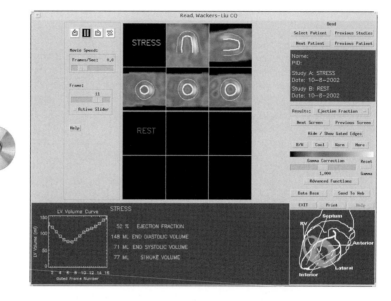

**Fig. 10-36.** WLCQ. Display of stress ECG-gated SPECT and computed endocardial edges for regional wall motion analysis and calculation of LVEF. In this patient LVEF is preserved at 52%, with anteroapical dyskinesis and anteroseptal hypokinesis. In addition the motion of the septum is paradoxical due to prior cardiac surgery. The end diastolic volume of 146 mL is relatively large.

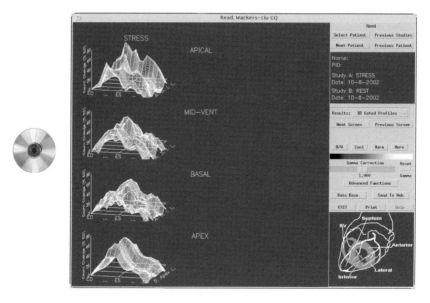

**Fig. 10-37.** WLCQ. Three-dimensional thickening profiles. In order to judge the quality of an ECG-gated SPECT study, in particular to recognize technical gating problems, inspection of the count recovery or thickening curves is useful.

Table 10-2
Comparative Characterization of Abnormal SPECT Results[a]

| Defect size | Small | Moderate | Large |
|---|---|---|---|
| Vascular territories | ≤ 1 | 1–2 | 2 or 3 |
| SSS* | 4–8 | 9–13 | >13 |
| Polar maps (% of LV)[+] | <10% | 10–20% | >20% |
| Circumf. Profile(% of LV)[#] | <5% | 5–10% | >10% |

[a]Modified from Wintergreen Panel Summaries (8).
*Summed stress score.
[+]Compared with Gender-matched normal file and reflects extent only.
[#]Circumferential profiles: based on Yale-CQ: Sum of defects in 36 interpolated slices. Compared to normal data files and incorporates both extent and severity.

## COMPARATIVE QUANTIFICATION OF SPECT IMAGES

Stress and rest myocardial perfusion abnormalities may be expressed as a percentage of left ventricular volume or as summed stress scores. One should be aware that defect size calculated using one method differs from that calculated by other methods. (See Table 10-2.)

## IMPORTANCE OF QUANTITATIVE IMAGE ANALYSIS

Reliable quantification of myocardial perfusion images, by any method, is extremely important and should be used for the following reasons:

- Quantification provides greater confidence in interpretation. Graphic display of relative count distribution, compared to a normal database, serves as an objective and consistent "second observer." The normal database serves as a consistent "benchmark" against which images are compared.
- Quantification provides enhanced intra- and interobserver interpretive reproducibility.
- Quantification provides a reproducible means of measuring the degree of abnormality. This is important since it is well established that the

---

(Fig. 10–37. *continued*) The figure shows families of thickening curves for apical, mid-ventricular, and basal short axis slices, and the apex (derived form horizontal long-axis slice). The Y-axis shows counts normalized to end-diastolic (ED) counts. The three-dimensional display shows the increase in count in systole (ES) and decrease in ED as circumferential profiles from anterior (A), septum (S), inferior (I), and lateral (L) wall. In a gated SPECT study with good ECG-synchronization, the thickening profiles start and end at the same count level. Thickening curves can thus be used as a method to recognize technical ECG-gating problems.

more abnormal a myocardial perfusion image, the poorer is patient outcome.

• Quantification of rest left ventricular ejection fraction from myocardial perfusion images provides additional important prognostic information *(9,10)*.

In our view, quantitative analysis is complementary to visual analysis. Interpretation should start with visual inspection of images using the following systematic approach:

1. Visual inspection of the unprocessed rotating planar images.
2. Visual analysis of reconstructed SPECT slices in three orthogonal cuts. Images should be inspected for overall quality and the presence of possible artifacts.
3. Quantitative display then serves to confirm and enhance the visual impression.

Quantitative analysis generally should not necessarily be expected to provide entirely new information. However, quantitative analysis may frequently be helpful clinically in adding a level of certainty in differentiating equivocal image features from abnormal or normal studies. We refer to this process as "quantitative analysis with visual overread."

## SELECTED BIBLIOGRAPHY

1. Port SC (ed) (1999). Imaging guidelines for nuclear cardiology procedures, part II. *J Nucl Cardiol* 6:G47–G84.
2. American Heart Association, American College of Cardiology, and Society of Nuclear Medicine (1992). Standardization of cardiac tomographic imaging. *Circulation* 86:338–339.
3. American Heart Association Writing Group on Myocardial Segmentation and Registration of Cardiac Imaging. Cerqueira MD, Weissman NJ, Dilsizian V, et al. (2002). Standardized myocardial segmentation and nomenclature for tomographic imaging of the heart. *Circulation* 105:539–542, *J Nucl Cardiol* 9:240–245.
4. Germano G, Kavanagh PB, Waechter P, et al. (2000). A new algorithm for the quantification of myocardial perfusion SPECT I: technical principles and reproducibility. *J Nucl Med* 41:712–719.
5. Germano G, Kiat H, et al. (1995). Automatic quantification of ejection fraction from gated myocardial perfusion SPECT. *J Nucl Med* 36:2138–2147.
6. Faber TL, Cooke CD, Folks RD, et al. (1999). Left ventricular function and perfusion images: an integrated method. *J Nucl Med* 40:650.
7. Liu YH, Sinusas AJ, DeMan P, et al. (1999). Quantification of SPECT myocardial perfusion images: methodology and validation of the method. *J Nucl Cardiol* 6:190.
8. Iskandrian AE (1999). Risk assessment of stable patients (panel III). In: Wintergreen panel summaries. *J Nucl Cardiol* 6:93–155.
9. Berman DS, Hachamovitch RH, Kiat H, et al. (1993). Incremental value of prognostic testing in patients with known or suspected ischemic heart disease: a basis for optimal utilization of single-photon emission computed tomography. *J Am Coll Cardiol* 6:665.

10. Vanzetto G, Ormezzano O, Fagret D, et al. (1999). Long term additive prognostic value of thallium-201 myocardial perfusion imaging over clinical and exercise stress test in low-to-intermediate risk patients. Study in 1,137 patients with 6 year-follow-up. *Circulation* 100:1521.

# 11 Display and Analysis of Planar Myocardial Perfusion Images

The display and nomenclature of nuclear cardiology images has been standardized. The analysis of nuclear cardiology images should follow a systematic approach and sequence as outlined in the Imaging Guidelines for Nuclear Cardiology Procedures, Part 2 *(1)* (on line: www.asnc.org; menu: library and resources: guidelines and standards).

## DISPLAY OF PLANAR IMAGES

For interpretation, planar stress-rest myocardial perfusion images are best displayed on computer screen side-by-side, i.e., either paired view-by-view (**Fig. 11-1**) or paired side-by-side (**Fig. 11-2**) as a complete three-view study. For planar images a linear gray scale is preferred over color display.

### *Breast Markers*

In order to recognize breast tissue attenuation, simultaneous display of breast markers may be useful (**Fig. 11-3**).

The Tl-201 images on the left in **Fig. 11-3** show apparent anteroseptal and anterolateral defects in the LAO1 (stress) and LAO2 (redistribution) views. The stress ANT1 view is normal, but the ANT2 redistribution view shows an apparent anterior wall defect. The appearance of the defects suggests breast attenuation. On the LAO2 small angle scatter can be noted (white linear pattern at the apex of the left ventricle). The breast marker images confirm this suspicion. The location of the breast markers on LAO1 and LAO2 match well with the boundary of the apparent anteroseptal and anterolateral defect. On the ANT1 view the contour of the breast is well above the heart (no attenuation) whereas on the ANT2 view the location of the breast marker matches with the anterior defect.

From: *Contemporary Cardiology: Nuclear Cardiology, The Basics*
F. J. Th. Wackers, W. Bruni, and B. L. Zaret © Humana Press Inc., Totowa, NJ

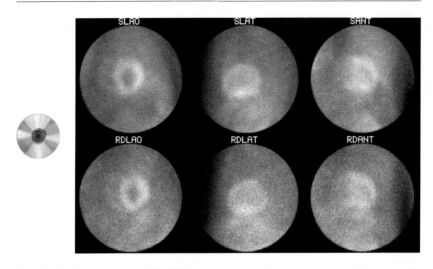

**Fig. 11-1.** Planar exercise Tl-201 images in view-by-view display. Exercise (S) images on top; rest (R) images on the bottom. There is mildly increased lung uptake and a reversible anteroseptal myocardial perfusion defect.

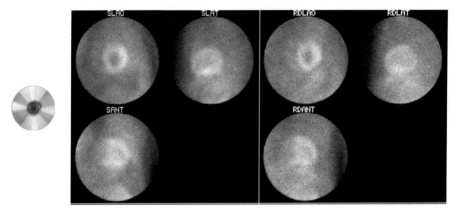

**Fig. 11-2.** Same planar exercise Tl-201 images as in Fig. 11-1 in side-by side display. Exercise (S) images on the left; rest (R) images on the right.

## ANALYSIS OF PLANAR IMAGES

Nomenclature and segmentation of planar myocardial perfusion imaging has been standardized in the Imaging Guidelines for Nuclear Cardiology Procedures, Part 2 *(1)* (on line: www.asnc.org; menu: library and resources: guidelines and standards), and are shown in **Figs. 11-4** and **11-5**.

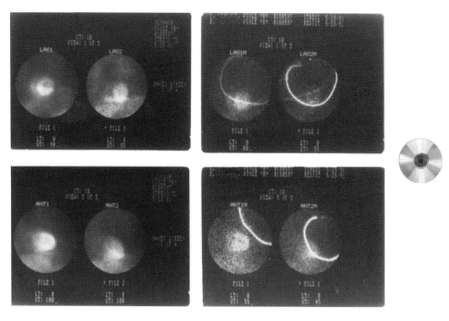

**Fig. 11-3.** Planar Tl-201 images (left) with breast markers (right).

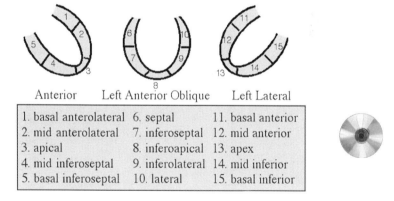

Anterior        Left Anterior Oblique        Left Lateral

| | | |
|---|---|---|
| 1. basal anterolateral | 6. septal | 11. basal anterior |
| 2. mid anterolateral | 7. inferoseptal | 12. mid anterior |
| 3. apical | 8. inferoapical | 13. apex |
| 4. mid inferoseptal | 9. inferolateral | 14. mid inferior |
| 5. basal inferoseptal | 10. lateral | 15. basal inferior |

**Fig. 11-4.** Standardized segmentation and nomenclature for planar myocardial perfusion images. (Reproduced with permission from ref. *1*.)

## QUANTITATIVE ANALYSIS

A number of validated commercial and noncommercial software packages are available for quantification of planar myocardial perfusion [CEQUAL *(2)*, University of Virginia *(3)*, and Yale University *(4)*]. Because of the current predominance of SPECT imaging in clinical practice, these software packages are no longer being developed.

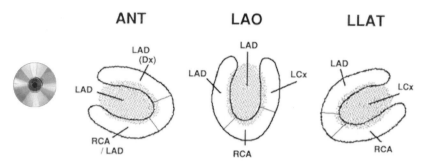

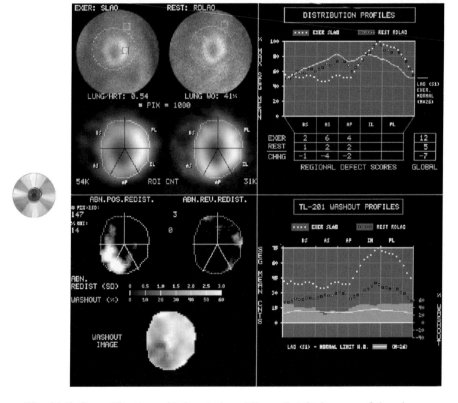

**Fig. 11-5.** Assignment of coronary artery territories on planar myocardial perfusion images. The shaded areas represent the projection of activity emanating from the facing walls overlying the left ventricular cavity. (LAD= left anterior descending coronary artery; Dx= diagonal coronary artery; LCx= left circumflex coronary artery; RCA= right coronary artery).

**Fig. 11-6.** Quantification of left anterior oblique (LAO) images of the planar Tl-201 images shown in Figs. 11-1 and 11-2. The top left panel shows raw LAO images with an elliptical region of interest (ROI) for interpolative background

The basic principles of planar quantification are similar for each of these software packages. Raw planar projection images are corrected for differences in background activity on rest and stress images by the application of interpolative background subtraction.

Normalized relative radiotracer uptake in the background subtracted left ventricular images is subsequently quantitatively compared with normal data files. Relative radiotracer uptake on planar images can be displayed in different ways *(2–4)*. In our laboratory we preferred circumferential count distribution profiles *(4)*. The size of myocardial perfusion defects can be expressed as percentage of the total potentially visualized normal left ventricle.

## EXAMPLE OF QUANTIFICATION OF PLANAR IMAGES

**Figures 11-6–11-8** show representative screen captures of quantification of exercise-delayed Tl-201 images of a patient with a reversible anteroseptal defect (shown in **Figs. 11-1** and **11-2**) using software developed in our laboratory *(4)*.

---

(**Fig. 11-6.** *continued*) subtraction and small square ROIs for lung/heart (HRT) ratio calculation. Lung/HRT ratio is abnormal at 0.54. Below in the same left top panel are the resulting background-corrected LAO images. On the top right are circumferential count profiles (exercise, white dots; rest, black dots) for quantification of defect size, displayed against the lower limit of normal Tl-201 uptake (white curve). Defect reversibility is quantified in the septal area (exercise defect is 12 and rest defect is 5). The lower right panel shows a graphic display of regional Tl-201 washout. Tl-201 washout is low in the septal region. The lower left panel shows functional images. In the top left image (ABN.POS.REDIST.), the background-corrected exercise image is subtracted pixel-by-pixel from the background-corrected rest image. The difference between the two images (=defect reversibility) is displayed as positive values in the septal area. To the right of this image (ABN.REV.REDIST), the rest image is subtracted from the exercise image. If reverse redistribution was present, this would show as positive values. The bottom image displays Tl-201 washout on a pixel-by-pixel basis. The darker area in the inferoseptal region indicates low washout.

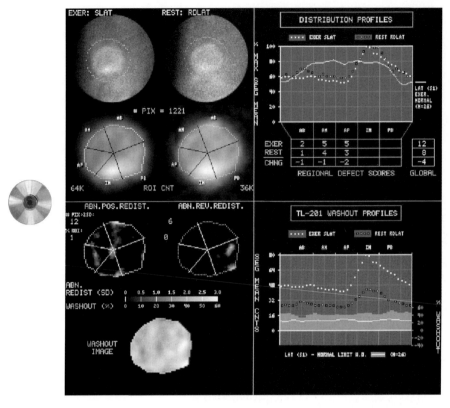

**Fig. 11-7.** Quantification of left lateral (LAT) images of the planar Tl-201 images shown in Figs. 11-1 and 11-2. The same quantification method described in Fig. 11-6 is used. A large fixed anterior wall defect is present.

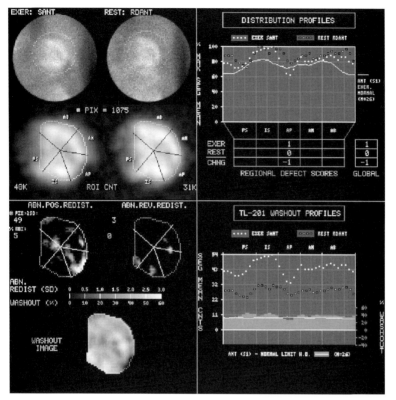

**Fig. 11-8.** Quantification of anterior (ANT) images of the planar Tl-201 images shown in Figs. 11-1 and 11-2. The same quantification method described in Fig. 11-6 is used. Except for a small apical defect, no quantifiable myocardial perfusion defect is present. Summary of quantitative analysis of three planar Tl-201 images (Figs. 11-6–11-8): Abnormal Tl-201 exercise-redistribution images with abnormally increased lung uptake after exercise and a large partially reversible anteroseptal myocardial perfusion defect.

## SELECTED BIBLIOGRAPHY

1. Port SC (ed) (1999). Imaging guidelines for nuclear cardiology procedures, part II. *J Nucl Cardiol* 6:G47.
2. Garcia E, Maddahi J, Berman D, et al. (1981). Space/time quantification of thallium-201 myocardial scintigraphy. *J Nucl Med* 22:309–317.
3. Watson DD, Campbell NP, Read EK, Gibson RS, Teates CD, Beller GA. (1981). Spatial and temporal quantitation of plane thallium myocardial images. *J Nucl Med* 22:577–584.
4. Wackers FJTh, Fetterman RC, Mattera JA, Clements JP (1985). Quantitative planar thallium-201 stress scintigraphy: a critical evaluation of the method. *Semin Nucl Med* 15:46–66.

# 12 Display and Analysis of Planar Equilibrium Angiocardiography

The display and nomenclature of nuclear cardiology images has been standardized. The analysis of nuclear cardiology images should follow a systematic approach and sequence as outlined in the Imaging Guidelines for Nuclear Cardiology Procedures, Part 2 *(1)* (on line: www.asnc.org; menu: library and resources: guidelines and standards).

## DISPLAY OF PLANAR ERNA IMAGES

It is standard that multiple views are displayed simultaneously in *cine or movie* format *(2)*. Multiple view planar ERNA images are best displayed simultaneously on a computer screen as endless loop movies. For planar ERNA images a linear gray scale is preferred over color display. The best speed to view ERNA movies is 10 frames/s. In order to be able to appreciate the morphology and function of the entire heart and great vessels, the gains of gamma camera should be set such that a normal heart occupies about one-quarter to one-third of the FOV. (See **Fig. 12-1.**)

## INTERPRETATION

The interpretation of ERNA images should follow a systematic approach *(2)*:
**Inspection of overall quality of images**

1. Size of the heart, right and left ventricle.
2. Size and contraction of right atrium.
3. Size and contraction of right ventricle.
4. Size of pulmonary artery.
5. Size and contraction of left atrium.
6. Size and contraction of left ventricle.
7. Size and morphology of ascending and descending aorta.

From: *Contemporary Cardiology: Nuclear Cardiology, The Basics*
F. J. Th. Wackers, W. Bruni, and B. L. Zaret © Humana Press Inc., Totowa, NJ

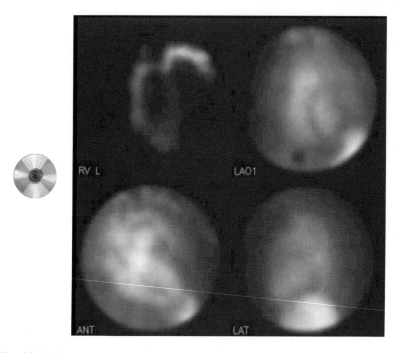

**Fig. 12-1.** Computer screen display of simultaneous movie display of planar ERNA images in left anterior oblique (LAO), anterior (ANT), and left lateral (LAT) views. In addition ECG-gated first pass angiocardiography for assessment of the right ventricle is displayed on the top left. The gains of the gamma camera were appropriately tuned so that the heart occupies about one-third of the field of view.

Interpretation of ERNA images is, with the exception of ejection fraction, largely based on visual analysis (**Figs. 12-2** and **12-3**). Overall quality of the study is determined by adequate labeling of red blood cells, the patient's weight, and counts emanating from the cardiac chambers. Although high labeling efficiency is important, free Tc-99m-pertechnetate usually is trapped in the thyroid gland and stomach mucosa and does not interfere with image interpretation. The most important problem is in obese patients in whom scattered photons significantly degrade image quality.

## *Statistical Accuracy of Ejection Fraction*

The accuracy of calculated right ventricular (RV) and left ventricular (LV) ejection fraction (EF) is dependent on count statistics. However, the lower the EF, the greater the counts required for optimal calculation.

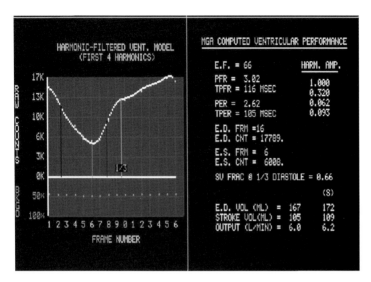

**Fig. 12-2.** Computer screen capture of normal ERNA. The left ventricular volume curve (left) shows a normal appearance. There is some count drop-off in the last frame due to respiratory heart rate variability. On the right are quantitative results of volume curve analysis. Left ventricular ejection fraction (EF) is normal at 66%. End diastolic (ED) counts (CNT) are excellent (17,789) ensuring good statistical reliability. Peak filling rate (PFR) is normal at 3.82 EDvolume/s. The ED volume (VOL) is at the upper limit of normal at 167 mL.

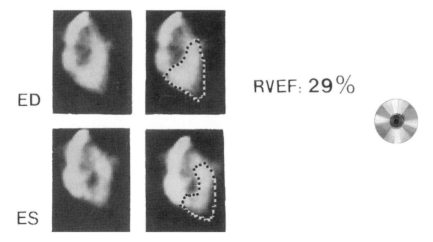

**Fig. 12-3.** Processed ECG-gated first pass angiocardiography. The end diastolic (ED) and end systolic (ES) frames are shown and the manually drawn regions of interest. RVEF is abnormal at 29%.

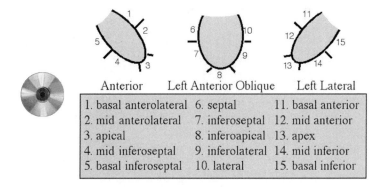

| Anterior | Left Anterior Oblique | Left Lateral |
|---|---|---|
| 1. basal anterolateral | 6. septal | 11. basal anterior |
| 2. mid anterolateral | 7. inferoseptal | 12. mid anterior |
| 3. apical | 8. inferoapical | 13. apex |
| 4. mid inferoseptal | 9. inferolateral | 14. mid inferior |
| 5. basal inferoseptal | 10. lateral | 15. basal inferior |

**Fig. 12-4.** Standardized segmentation and nomenclature for planar equilibrium ventriculography. (Reproduced with permission from ref. *1*.)

We use the following rule of thumb:

- If LVEF is normal (> 0.50), at least 5,000 counts are required in the background corrected LV end diastolic region of interest (ROI).
- If LVEF is moderately abnormal (< 0.40), at least 20,000 counts are required in the background corrected end diastolic ROI.

## NOMENCLATURE OF ERNA

The nomenclature and segmentation (**Fig. 12-4**) of planar ERNA imaging have been standardized in the Imaging Guidelines for Nuclear Cardiology Procedures, Part 2 *(1)* (on line: www.asnc.org; menu: library and resources: guidelines and standards).

## SELECTED BIBLIOGRAPHY

1. Port SC (ed.) (1999). Imaging guidelines for nuclear cardiology procedures, part 2. *J Nucl Cardiol* 6:G47–G84.
2. Wackers FJTh (1996). Equilibrium radionuclide angiocardiography. In Gerson MC (ed.), *Cardiac Nuclear Medicine*, 3rd Edition, Chapter 11=. McGraw-Hill, New York, NY.

# 13 Display and Analysis of SPECT Equilibrium Radionuclide Angiocardiography

At time of this writing SPECT ERNA is not routinely performed in most nuclear cardiology laboratories. Consequently, no standards have been set for display and analysis of SPECT ERNA. It seems reasonable to use a similar approach for SPECT ERNA as for SPECT myocardial perfusion imaging.

The display of ERNA SPECT should include at a minimum:

1. Rotating planar projection images.
2. Reconstructed static slices.
3. Movie display of selected multiple ECG-gated slices: vertical long axis, short axis and horizontal long axis.
4. Left ventricular volume curve.

Interpretation of SPECT ERNA images should follow a similar systematic approach and quality control as described for SPECT myocardial perfusion imaging.

## DISPLAY OF SPECT ERNA

Static reconstructed SPECT slices should be displayed using the same planes as for SPECT myocardial perfusion images (**Fig. 13-1**).

## MOVIE DISPLAY

The uniqueness of SPECT ERNA is that ECG-gated blood pool movies can be analyzed at any desired plane in one of three conventional tomographic cuts (**Figs. 13-2, 13-3**). This allows for detailed analysis of

From: *Contemporary Cardiology: Nuclear Cardiology, The Basics*
F. J. Th. Wackers, W. Bruni, and B. L. Zaret © Humana Press Inc., Totowa, NJ

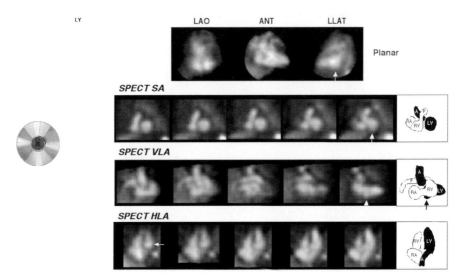

**Fig. 13-1.** Display of SPECT ERNA. The reconstructed static slices of a patient with an inferobasal aneurysm (arrow) are shown. At the top are conventional planar images of the same patient.

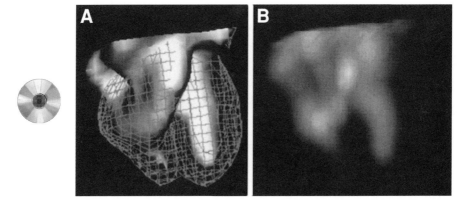

**Fig. 13-2.** Three-dimensional surface-shades **(A)** and volume-rendered **(B)** SPECT ERNA in long-axis projection. End diastolic birdcage **(A)** is used as reference for assessment of regional wall motion *(1)*. Reproduced with permission from ref. *1*.

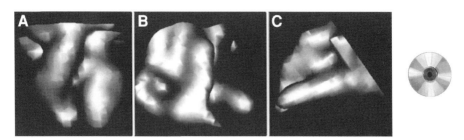

**Fig. 13-3.** Three views of surface-shaded and three-dimensional rendering of SPECT ERNA in long-axis **(A)**, anterior **(B)**, and lateral **(C)** equivalents to planar imaging *(1)*. Reproduced with permission from ref. *1*.

regional wall motion without superimposition of other cardiac structures. In addition, global and regional function can be inspected on three dimensional volume-rendered movie display. The user is able to rotate the heart in space on the computer screen and view the contraction of the heart from any desired angle. Thus, in addition to left ventricular function, right ventricular function can be analyzed as well.

## LEFT VENTRICULAR FUNCTION

The methodology for the calculation of left ventricular ejection fraction from SPECT ERNA is not well standardized. In general ERNA SPECT LVEF correlates well with that obtained by planar ERNA, although the value for LVEF is usually higher.

## SELECTED BIBLIOGRAPHY

1. Groch MW, DePuey EG, Belzberg AC, et al. (2001). Planar imaging versus gated blood-pool SPECT for assessment of ventricular performance: a multicenter study. *J Nucl Med* 42:1773–1779.

# 14 Artifacts and Technical Problems in Cardiac Imaging

When interpreting nuclear cardiology images, one should always consider the possibility of artifacts or other technical problems that may interfere with image quality. Artifacts are not unexpected in conventional SPECT imaging. During the process of external detection of relatively low-energy photons emanating from inside the body, tissue attenuation, noncardiac uptake, and motion may distort images.

Examples of artifacts and other problems, their recognition and correction are discussed in this chapter and on the CD Rom that accompanies this book.

Various artifacts and problems will be addressed in the temporal sequence one might encounter them in the course of interpreting nuclear cardiology images.

## SPECT MYOCARDIAL PERFUSION IMAGING

### *Rotating Images*

Inspection of the rotating planar projection images (**Fig. 14-1**, on CD Rom) is always the first step of interpretation, because these images may provide important clues for problems or artifacts to be anticipated during analysis of reconstructed SPECT images.

### Low Counts (Figs. 14-2 to 14-4)

One of the most important parameters affecting image quality is count density. Low count density can be suspected readily from the visual appearance of the rotating planar projection images (**Fig. 14-2**, on CD Rom). Low count studies have an overall "noisy" appearance and the

From: *Contemporary Cardiology: Nuclear Cardiology, The Basics*
F. J. Th. Wackers, W. Bruni, and B. L. Zaret © Humana Press Inc., Totowa, NJ

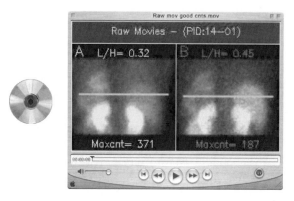

**Fig. 14-1.** Cine display of rotating planar projection images. In this, and all following movies of projection images, the stress study is on the left and the rest study is on the right. The horizontal white line serves as a reference mark and is placed by the technologist approximately at the level of the left ventricular apex. The most convenient display speed for inspecting these images is at 10 frames/second. The lung/heart ratio (L/H) is displayed, as is the maximal count density/pixel within the left ventricle. Studies with maximal cardiac counts/ pixel < 100 are of suboptimal quality. The rotating projection images should always be viewed before analysis of reconstructed tomographic slices. The images should be inspected for patient motion, breast shadow and overall quality.

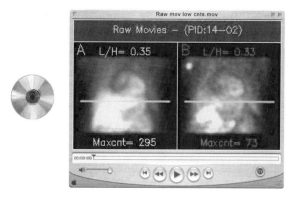

**Fig. 14-2.** Cine display of rotating planar projection images. The count density of the rest study as measured by maximal count/pixel within the left ventricle is low (73 counts). The stress study in contrast has excellent count density. One can expect the reconstructed tomographic slices of the rest study to be of sub-optimal quality.

heart is poorly visualized. Software developed in our laboratory displays maximal counts/pixel in the left ventricle on the rotating images screen.

Good quality SPECT images (**Fig. 14-4**) usually have > 150 maximal counts/pixel in the heart. Low count studies are often caused by patient obesity. It is helpful if the imaging worksheet for technologists contains

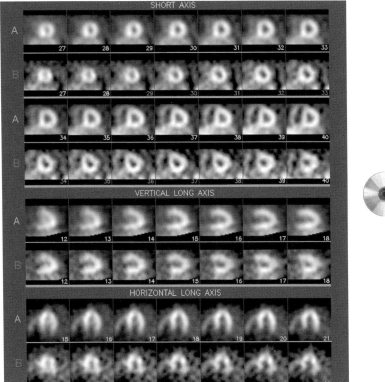

**Fig. 14-3.** Reconstructed SPECT slices of the raw projection data shown in Fig. 14-2. The display of reconstructed slices in this and other images follows ASNC standards. The short-axis (SA) slices are displayed on top, the vertical long-axis (VLA) slices in the middle, and the horizontal long-axis (HLA) slices on the bottom. The rows marked with "A" show the stress images and rows marked with "B" show rest images. The SA slices are displayed from apex (#27) to base (#40); the VLA slices are displayed from septum (#12) to lateral wall (#18); the HLA are displayed from inferior wall (#15) to anterior wall (#21). The suboptimal quality of the low-count rest images can be appreciated in comparison to the good quality stress images.

information about patient weight, chest circumference, and bra size (see page 71).

Low count density SPECT studies can be avoided in two ways: by increasing the injected dose or by increasing the imaging time. One can use patient weight or chest circumference as a guide for increasing these parameters (see Chapter 6, pages 63,64). Another practical method for avoiding low count studies involves the acquisition of a short (e.g., 15 s)

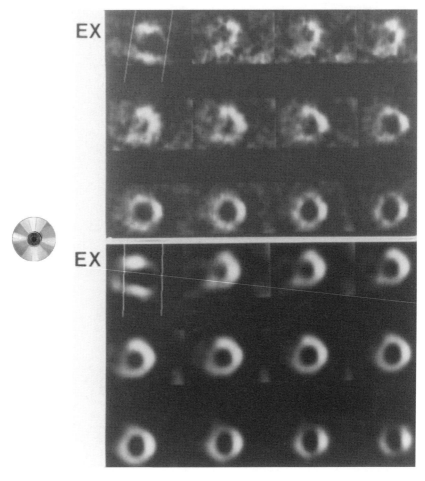

**Fig. 14-4.** Reconstructed SPECT slices of a patient with an anteroseptal and apical myocardial perfusion defect. The top study was acquired with Thallium-201 and is of suboptimal quality due to relatively low counts (max 87 cnts/pixel). The study was repeated with Tc-99m Sestamibi (bottom). This study is of excellent quality with high count density (256 cnts/pixel).

"scout" planar image prior to the start of SPECT acquisition. By comparing total counts in this image to "usual" count density in other patients, one may identify the potential for a low count study ahead of time and make appropriate adjustments. This preventive QA method is particularly recommended for Tl-201 SPECT imaging.

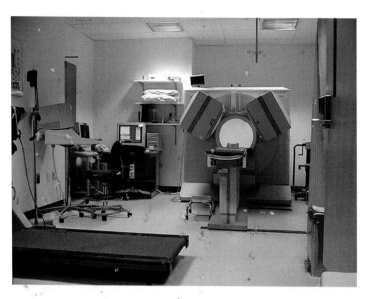

**Color Plate 1.** Nuclear cardiology imaging and stress facility. In the background are a triple-head gamma camera and computer. On the left in front is a motorized treadmill.

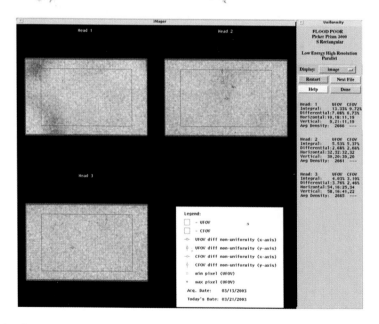

**Color Plate 2.** Daily uniformity floods of a triple-head gamma camera. Good uniformity is important for reliable detection of regional myocardial perfusion defects. This example shows daily quality control images. The flood of head 1 (upper left) shows several areas of severe non-uniformity (dark areas). Head 2 (upper right) shows only minor non-uniformity, whereas head 3 (bottom left) shows good uniformity. The gamma camera must be tuned-up by service before clinical imaging is performed.

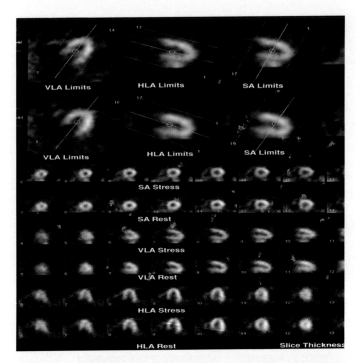

**Color Plate 3.** Example of correct slicing of the heart (top 2 rows) for obtaining cardiac tomographic slices (bottom 6 rows). The direction of slicing (green lines) must be parallel or perpendicular to the anatomical axes of the left ventricle.

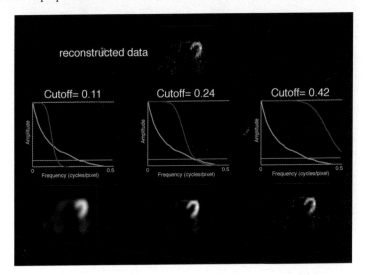

**Color Plate 4.** Effect of filtering cutoff on image quality. With a high cutoff value (right) significant noise is present in the image. In contrast using a low cutoff value (left) the image is markedly blurred. Appropriate selection of the filtering cutoff value should aim to achieve a balance between the two extremes, resulting in images of good diagnostic quality (middle).

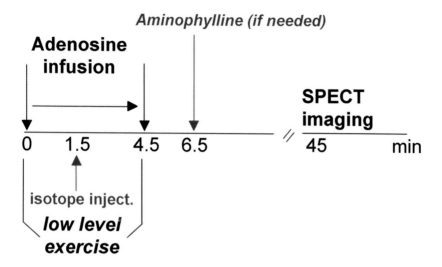

**Color Plate 5.** Short adenosine infusion protocol. Because of rapid onset of coronary vasodilation during adenosine infusion, the radiopharmaceutical can be injected shortly (1.5 min) after the start of infusion of adenosine. SPECT imaging is started after an interval of 45 min.

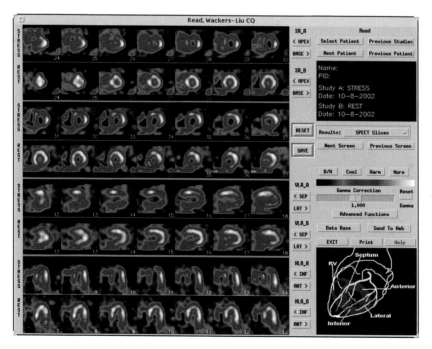

**Color Plate 6.** Tc-99m-sestamibi stress and rest single photon emission computed tomographic (SPECT) slices of a patient with severe anteroseptal and inferior ischemia. The stress images are markedly abnormal in the anteroseptal and inferior walls, whereas the rest images are normal.

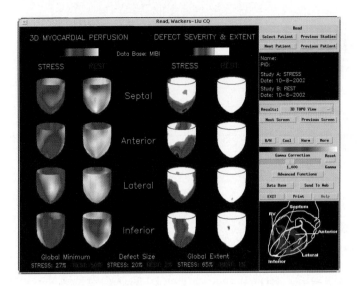

**Color Plate 7.** Three dimensional display of the SPECT slices in color plate 6. The three dimensional representation shows the septal, anterior, lateral, and inferior wall. The two sets of images on the left show relative radiopharmaceutical uptake on the stress (far left) and rest (near left) images. The dark-colored areas indicate decreased radiotracer uptake. The set of images on the right show radiotracer uptake relative to normal limits. The abnormal areas are displayed in color. The stress images are markedly abnormal in the apical anteroseptal and inferolateral regions, wheras the rest images are normal.

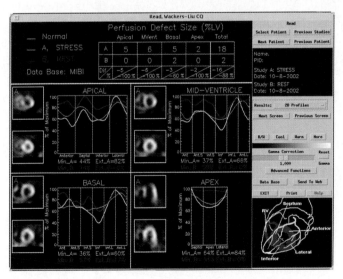

**Color Plate 8.** Quantification of the images in color plate 6 using circumferential count profile analysis. The yellow profiles represent the count distribution on the stress images, the red profiles represent count distribution on the rest images. The white curve is the lower limit of normal radiotracer uptake. Relative to the lower limit of normal, the stress defect is quantified to involve 18% of the left ventricle, which is a large abnormality. The rest study is near normal with a small residual defect of 2%.

## Low Counts

> *Recognition*
> Record count rate prior to start of acquisition in planar scout image.
> *Preventive measure*
> Adjust dose according to weight/chest circumference.
> Adjust acquisition time according to weight/chest circumference.
> *Corrective measure*
> Repeat imaging with longer imaging times.

## Motion (Figs. 14-5 to 14-19)

Patient motion may be up-and-down (Y-axis), or sideways (X-axis). Motion in the Z-axis is difficult to identify and to correct for. In addition to motion caused by the patient, there may be a gradual change in position of the heart itself within the chest, e.g., upward creep after a good exercise effort. Inspection of rotating planar projection images is important for the recognition of motion.

A simple and commonly used method for identifying patient motion or upward creep consists of the use of a *horizontal reference line* on the computer screen. Using such a line as a fixed reference, e.g., at the level of the apex, up-and-down motion of the heart can be readily recognized.

Another more sophisticated method involves the generation of a *sinogram* (**Fig. 14-5**) in which each horizontal row of pixels represents the summed counts of an entire projection image on the x-axis. Motion can be recognized by "breaks" in the smooth sinusoid pattern of inhomogeneous activity. A modification of the sinogram is the *linogram* in which each vertical column represent summed counts of the cardiac activity.

Most vendors supply motion correction software. Motion correction software does not always correct appropriately and must be used judiciously. Prevention of motion is the most effective way to avoid artifacts. One should take time to instruct patients about the importance of remaining still on the table and the use straps or hand holds to facilitate this.

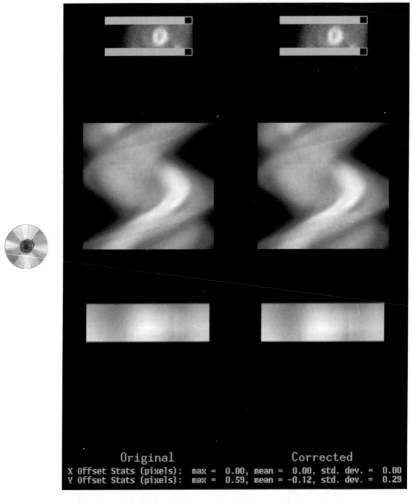

```
                Original                        Corrected
X Offset Stats (pixels):  max =  0.00, mean =  0.00, std. dev. =  0.00
Y Offset Stats (pixels):  max =  0.59, mean = -0.12, std. dev. =  0.29
```

**Fig. 14-5.** Normal sinogram. The simplest method to recognize patient motion is the horizontal reference line as shown in Fig 14-1. The sinogram as shown in this figure is another method. A normal sinogram shows smooth and continuous curves (sinusoids) of activity. Projecting all activity in one projection image on the X-axis creates this image. Owing to the rotating motion of the gamma camera, the location of projected counts at each stop moves in a sinusoid pattern. In this image the brightest activity are counts from the heart. As can be seen there are no breaks in the sinusoid pattern, indicating no patient motion. On the bottom the X and Y offsets are shown. In the absence of significant motion only minor corrections are made.

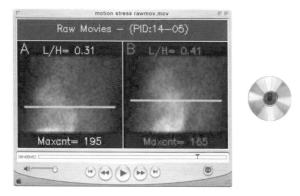

**Fig. 14-6.** Cine display of rotating planar projection images of a patient who moved during acquisition of the SPECT study. The heart can be seen "bouncing" on the left stress images, indicating marked patient motion. The stress study is not motion corrected. This can be concluded because the image itself is not moving. The rest study is apparently motion corrected as the projection images are moving up and down while rotating.

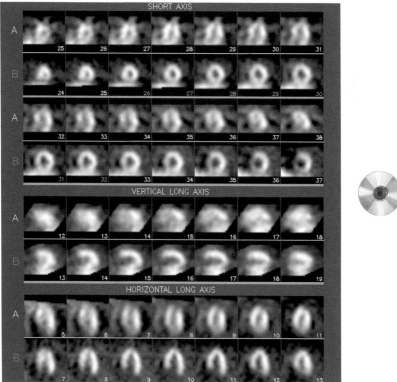

**Fig. 14-7.** Reconstructed slices of the study in 14-6. The motion-corrected rest study appears normal. However, the stress study shows marked distortion of the normal morphology of the heart in short axis slices and vertical and horizontal long axis slices. The stress study is uninterpretable.

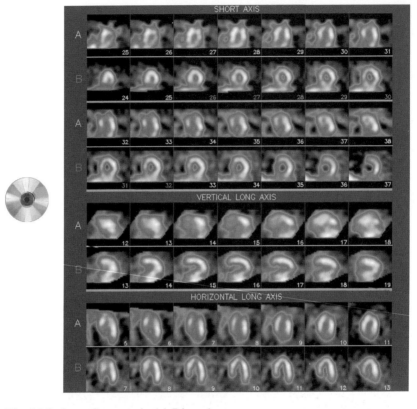

**Fig. 14-8.** Same figure as in 14-7 in color.

**Fig. 14-9.** (*Top right*) Cine display of rotating planar projection images of the same study as in Figs. 14-5 to 14-7. Motion correction is applied to both the stress and rest studies. Note the up-and-down motion of the projection images due to correction in the Y-axis. Although there is still some motion of the heart after correction, it is significantly less.

**Fig. 14-10.** (*Bottom right*) Motion-corrected reconstructed slices of the study in Figs. 14-5 to 14-7. The quality of the stress study is markedly improved. The motion-corrected stress study shows a very small reversible inferoapical defect. This is a good example of successful motion correction.

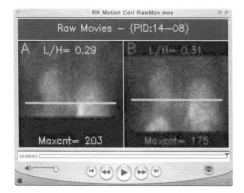

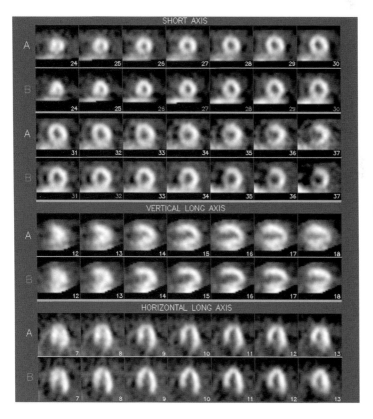

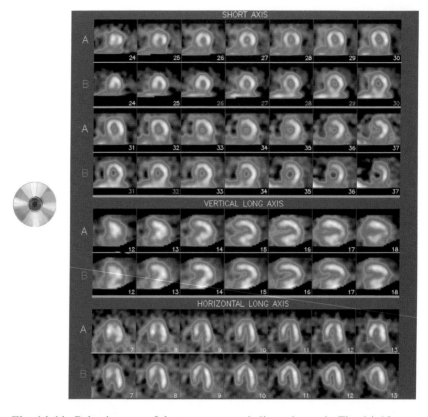

**Fig. 14-11.** Color images of the reconstructed slices shown in Fig. 14-10.

**Fig. 14-12.** (*Top right*) Sinogram (original [left] and motion-corrected [right]) of the patient study shown in Fig. 14-5 to 14-10. The corrected sinogram is by no means normal but greatly improved compared to the original one. The X and Y offset of pixels is shown on the bottom.

**Fig. 14-13.** (*Bottom right*) Cine display of rotating planar projection images of another patient who moved during acquisition of the SPECT study. The heart can be seen "bouncing" on the left stress images, indicating marked patient motion. In addition to up-and-down motion, there is also marked sideways motion in the anterior position. The stress study is not motion corrected as the image itself is not moving. The rest study is apparently motion corrected, as the projection images are moving up and down while rotating.

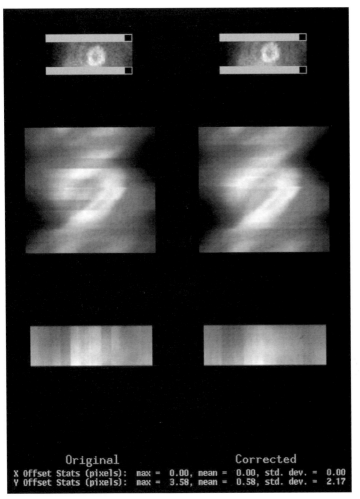

Original                              Corrected
X Offset Stats (pixels):   max =   0.00, mean =   0.00, std. dev. =   0.00
Y Offset Stats (pixels):   max =   3.58, mean =   0.58, std. dev. =   2.17

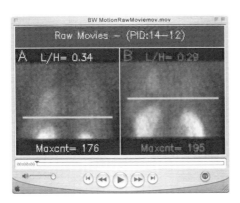

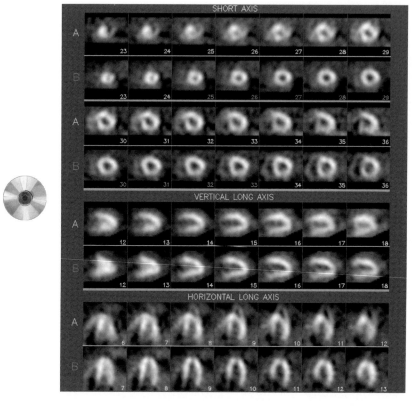

**Fig. 14-14.** Reconstructed slices of the study in 14-13. The motion-corrected rest study appears relatively normal. However, the stress study shows marked distortion of the normal morphology of the heart in short-axis slices and vertical and horizontal long-axis slices. The stress study is uninterpretable.

**Fig. 14-15.** (*Top right*) Same images as in Fig. 14-14 in color.

**Fig. 14-16.** (*Bottom right*) Cine display of rotating planar projection images of the same study as in Figs. 14-13 to 14-15. Motion correction is applied to both the stress and rest studies. Note the up-and-down motion of the projection images due to correction in the Y-axis. Although the up-and-down motion of the stress study is less, the sideways motion is still present. On the rest image motion correction was effective.

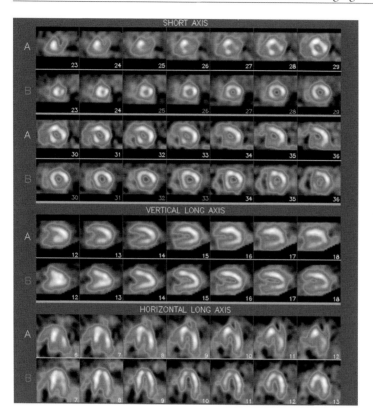

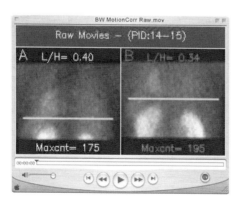

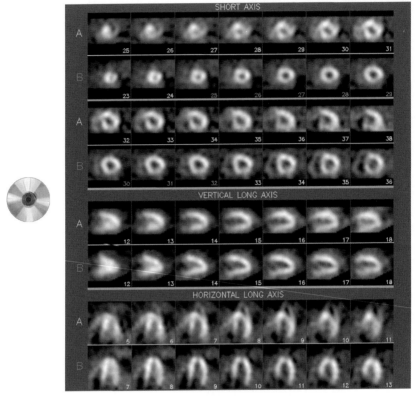

**Fig. 14-17.** Motion-corrected stress and rest reconstructed slices of the study shown in Figs. 14-13 to 14-15. Motion correction was not successful on the stress study. There is still marked distortion of normal morphology. The study remains uninterpretable. The rest study is successfully corrected for motion.

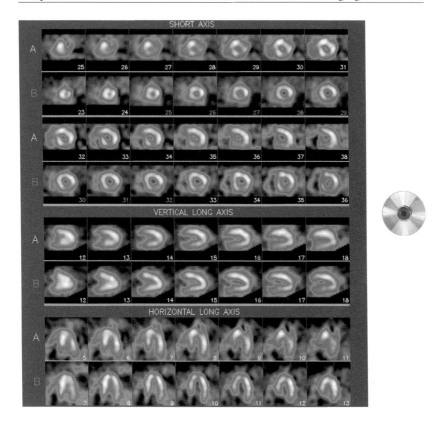

**Fig. 14-18.** Same images as in Fig. 14-17 in color.

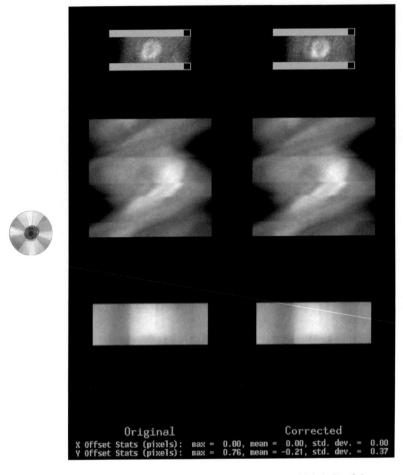

**Fig. 14-19.** Sinogram (original [left] and motion-corrected [right]) of the stress study shown in Figs. 14-13 to 14-18. The corrected sinogram is still markedly abnormal. The X and Y offset of pixels is shown on the bottom. The computer algorithm erroneously did not make correction for X-axis offset.

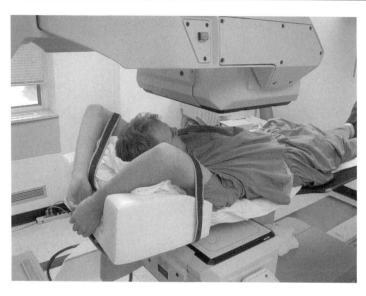

**Fig. 14-20.** For many patients it is difficult to keep still with the arms extended over the head. Velcro straps may be helpful in making this position more tolerable.

## MOTION ARTIFACT

*Recognition*
Horizontal reference line.
Sinogram.
Linogram.
*Preventive measure*
Explain to patients the importance of not moving and not falling asleep (snoring):
Position patient in comfortable position.
Immobilize arms with Velcro straps.
Delay stress imaging until 10–15 min after exercise to avoid upward creep.
*Corrective measure*
Apply motion-correction software.
Repeat imaging after better patient instruction and better immobilization with straps.

ᴀᴛᴛᴇɴᴜᴀᴛɪᴏɴ (Fɪɢ. **14-21** ᴛᴏ Fɪɢ. **14-40**)

imaging is performed with the patient in the supine position. In this position the dome of the left hemidiaphragm may attenuate photons emanating from the inferior wall of the left ventricle. Diaphragmatic attenuation can be suspected when the inferior wall *suddenly* disappears when going from left anterior oblique to left lateral angles on the rotating planar projection images.

Diaphragmatic attenuation can be demonstrated by acquiring two planar left lateral images: one with the patient *supine* and one with the patient on the *right-side decubitus* position *(1–3)* (**Fig. 14-25**). Inferior attenuation is present when the left lateral right decubitus is normal and the supine image shows an inferior wall defect. This occurs in about one-quarter of patients.

Inferior attenuation usually results in fixed myocardial perfusion defects mimicking infarction. ECG-gated SPECT has been very helpful in differentiating inferior attenuation from scar: if regional wall motion and thickening are normal in a region with a fixed inferior defect, the defect is likely caused by attenuation *(4)*.

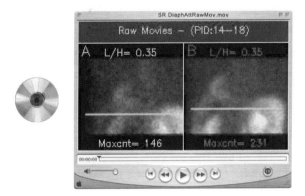

**Fig. 14-21.** Rotating planar projection images of a patient with inferior attenuation. Note how the inferior wall suddenly disappears on the stress and rest left lateral projection images.

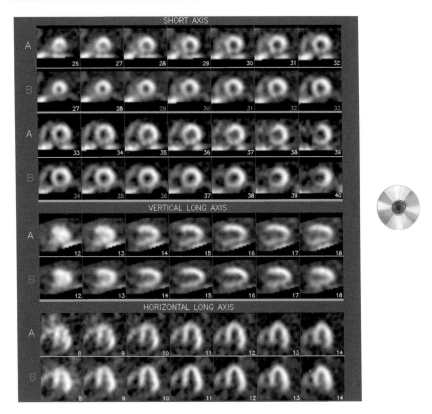

**Fig. 14-22.** Reconstructed tomographic slices of the images shown in Fig. 14-21. A fixed inferior myocardial perfusion defect is present.

Inferior attenuation can be avoided by performing SPECT imaging in a different position: right-side decubitus **(Fig. 14-25)**, upright sitting, and prone **(Fig. 14-32)**. In many centers imaging is repeated in prone position if inferior attenuation is suspected. Nevertheless, these methods have only limited utility: patient with inferior attenuation may also have coronary artery disease.

The only effective methodology to deal with nonuniform attenuation artifacts is to acquire images with effective attenuation correction *(5)*.

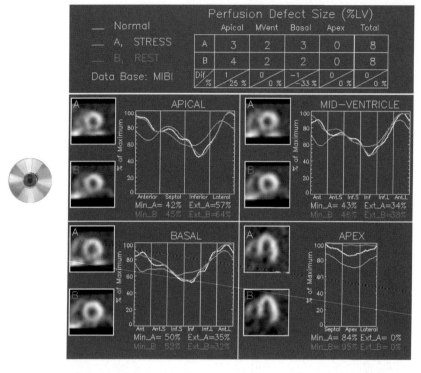

**Fig. 14-23.** Quantification of the SPECT slices in Fig. 14-22. The yellow curves represent the count distribution on the stress images and the red curves represent the rest images. The white curve represents the lower limit of normal radiotracer distribution. The stress and rest curves are below the lower limit of normal in the inferolateral walls in the apical, midventricular, and basal short axis slices. Note that the yellow and red curves are virtually identical, indicating a fixed myocardial perfusion abnormality due to either scar or attenuation. In the table at the top the results of computer quantification are shown. The total stress and rest defect size is moderate and involves 8% of the left ventricle.

---

**Fig. 14-24.** (*Top right*) Movie display of ECG-gated SPECT of images shown in Fig. 14-22. Note that the wall motion and thickening of the inferior wall (location of fixed defect) is normal. This suggests that the fixed defect may be artifactual and due to attenuation.

**Fig. 14-25.** (*Bottom right*) Planar left-lateral images of the patient whose reconstructed SPECT images were shown in Fig. 14-22. Planar images were acquired in supine position (top) and in right side decubitus position (bottom). One can appreciate that the planar images on the bottom are normal with good visualization of the inferior wall, whereas on the supine images, in the position that SPECT was acquired, the inferior wall is practically absent due to attenuation. The constellation of findings on rotating images, gated images, and planar images all confirm the presence of inferior attenuation.

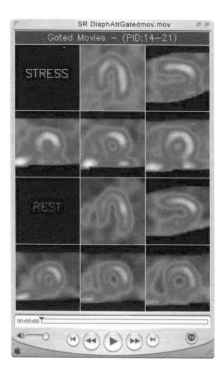

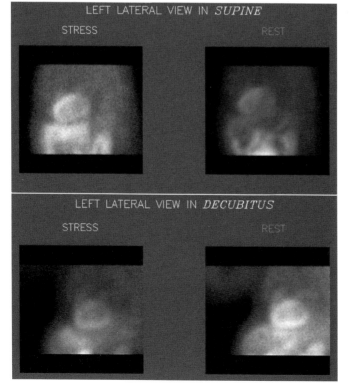

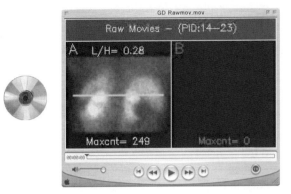

**Fig. 14-26.** Rotating planar projection images of another patient with inferior attenuation. Note again how the inferior wall suddenly disappears on the stress left lateral projection images.

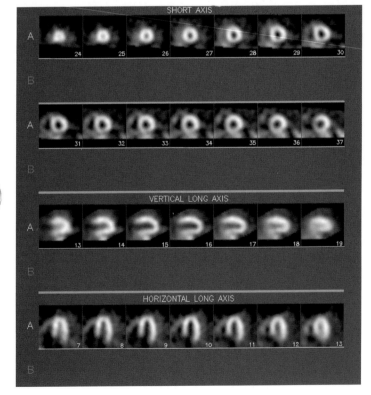

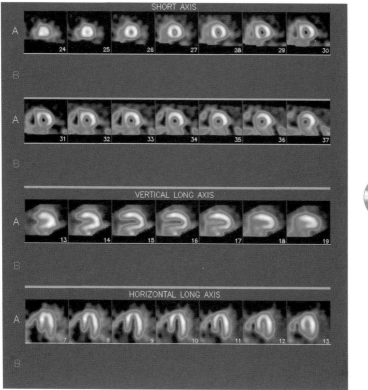

**Fig. 14-28.** Same images as in Fig. 14-27 in color. The decreased uptake in the inferior wall is better appreciated.

---

**Fig. 14-27.** (*Bottom left*) Reconstructed tomographic slices of the images shown in Fig. 14-26. Mild decreased uptake in the inferior wall is noted.

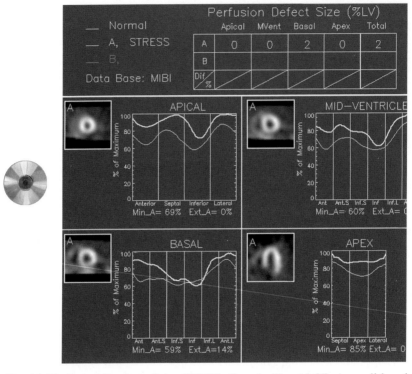

**Fig. 14-29.** Quantification of the SPECT slices in Fig. 14-27. A small basal inferior wall perfusion defect (2%) is present.

**Fig. 14-30.** (*Top right*) Planar left lateral images of the patient in Fig. 14-27. In supine position there is inferobasal defect, which is not present on the image acquired in the right-side decubitus position. This suggests the presence of inferior attenuation.

**Fig. 14-31.** (*Bottom right*) Movie display of ECG-gated SPECT of images in Fig. 14-27. Note that wall motion and thickening of the inferior wall are normal. This suggests that the small basal defect may be due to attenuation.

LEFT LATERAL VIEW IN *SUPINE*

STRESS

LEFT LATERAL VIEW IN *DECUBITUS*

STRESS

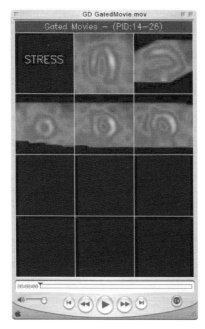

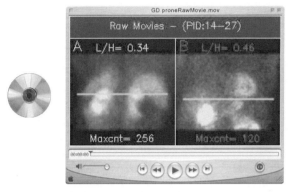

**Fig. 14-32.** Rotating planar projection images of the patient, whose images were shown in Figs. 14-26 to 14-31. The patient had repeat imaging in prone position. The supine stress images are displayed on the left; the prone stress images are displayed on the right. Note that because of the different patient position the images rotate in opposite directions.

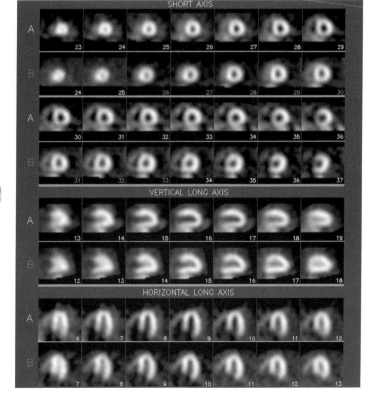

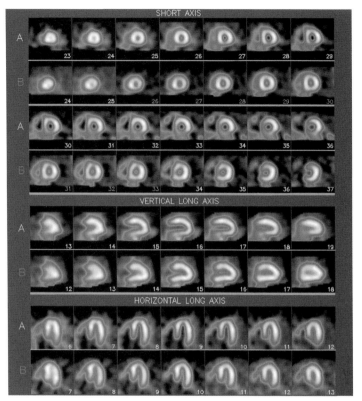

**Fig. 14-34.** Same images as in Fig. 14-33 in color.

**Fig. 14-33.** (*Bottom Left*) Reconstructed tomographic slices of the images in Fig. 14-32. The stress *supine* images are shown in rows "A"; whereas the *prone* images are shown in rows "B." The small inferior defect present on the supine images is not present on the prone images.

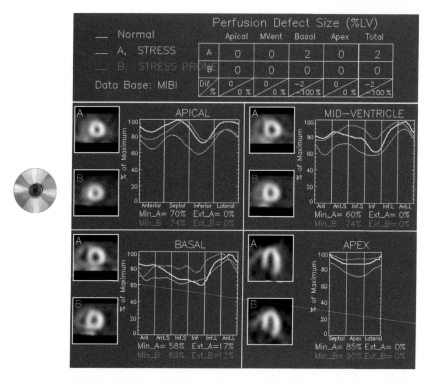

**Fig. 14-35.** Quantification of the SPECT images in Figs. 14-28 (supine) and 14-33 (prone). The yellow curves represent the circumferential count distribution profiles on the supine images, whereas the red curves represent that on the prone images. It can be appreciated that in the mid ventricular and basal slices inferior attenuation is significantly less in prone position than in supine position.

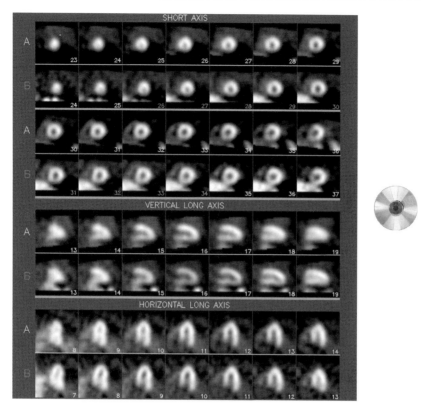

**Fig. 14-36.** Stress and rest reconstructed slices of another patient with probable inferior wall attenuation. The slices show a small fixed inferior defect. Supine and right-side decubitus planar left lateral images suggested attenuation of the inferior wall. Inferior wall thickening on gated SPECT was normal.

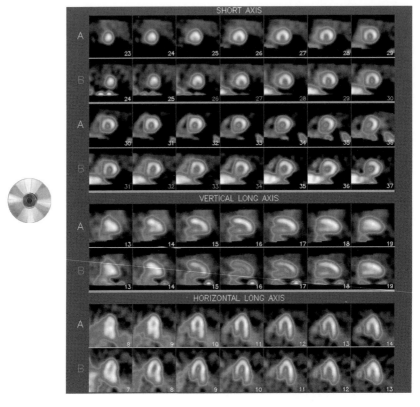

**Fig. 14-37.** Same images as in Fig. 14-36 in color.

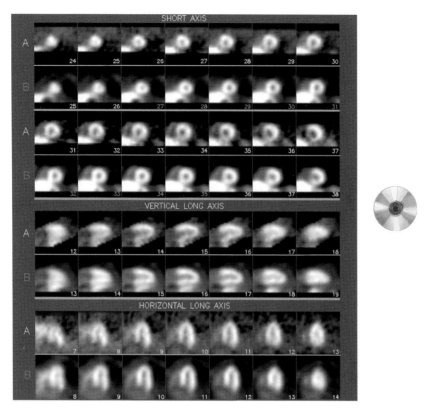

**Fig. 14-38.** Rest SPECT imaging (of study shown in Figs. 14-36 and 14-37) was performed with X-ray CT attenuation correction. Shown are the uncorrected images in rows "A" and attenuation-corrected images in rows "B." On the attenuation-corrected images radiotracer distribution is more homogeneous. There is no longer an inferior wall defect.

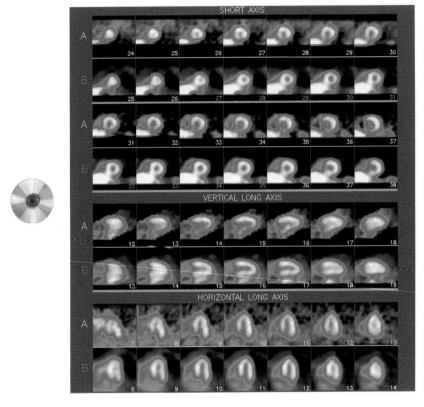

**Fig. 14-39.** Same images as in Fig. 14-38 in color.

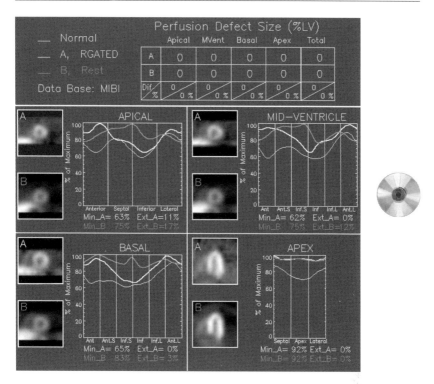

**Fig. 14-40.** Quantification of the images in Figs. 14-38 and 14-39. The yellow curves represent the circumferential count distribution profiles of the *uncorrected* images, whereas the red curves represent that of the *attenuation-corrected* images. It can be appreciated that radiotracer distribution is more homogeneous after attenuation correction.

## DIAPHRAGMATIC ATTENUATION

> *Recognition inferior attenuation*
> Compare planar left lateral images in supine and right-side decu-
> bitus position.
> *Preventive measure*
> Imaging in prone, upright, or right-side decubitus position.Normal
> regional wall motion and thickening on gated SPECT.
> *Corrective measure*
> Attenuation correction.

## BREAST ATTENUATION (FIG. 14-41 TO FIG. 14-46)

When interpreting SPECT images of women, the rotating planar projection images should always be scrutinized for breast attenuation. In
some obese men, upper chest attenuation may also occur.

On rotating images the breast can be recognized as a round shadow
that moves over the heart in the left anterior oblique and lateral positions.
It is helpful if the technologist records information about chest circumference and bra size on the imaging worksheet.

In contrast to the serious interpretative problems one can have on
*planar* images due to breast attenuation, breast attenuation on SPECT
images is often not a significant problem. Most of the time only a mild
fixed anterior defect may be present. *Because of possible change in
position of the breast on rest and stress images, the defect is not necessarily fixed.* In order to reduce variable attenuation by breast tissue,
stress and rest images must be acquired both with bras off or with bras
on. Again analysis of regional wall motion on ECG-gated SPECT has
been shown to be helpful in recognizing breast artifacts *(4)*.

Nevertheless, these methods have only limited utility: a patient with
anterior attenuation may also have coronary artery disease.

The only effective methodology to deal with nonuniform attenuation
artifacts is to acquire images with attenuation-correction *(5)*.

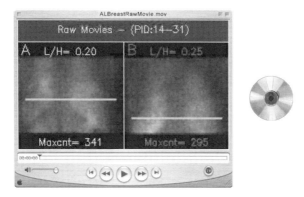

**Fig. 14-41.** Rotating planar projection images of a patient with large breasts. Chest circumference was 44 inches (112 cm) and bra cup size was DD. Note that both the right and left breasts can be seen as shadows that move over the screen. The left breast almost completely eclipses the heart.

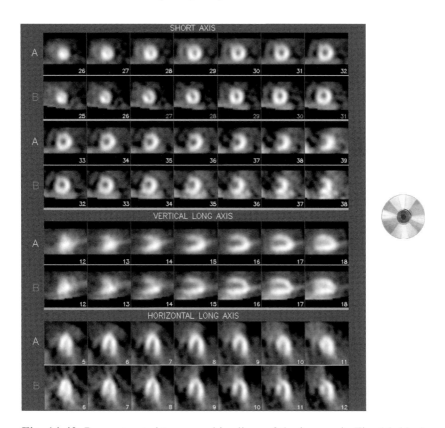

**Fig. 14-42.** Reconstructed tomographic slices of the images in Fig. 14-41. A moderate fixed anterior wall defect can be noted on the stress and rest images on short-axis and vertical long-axis slices. The "streaks" at the apex on the horizontal long axis slices may be due to breast tissue.

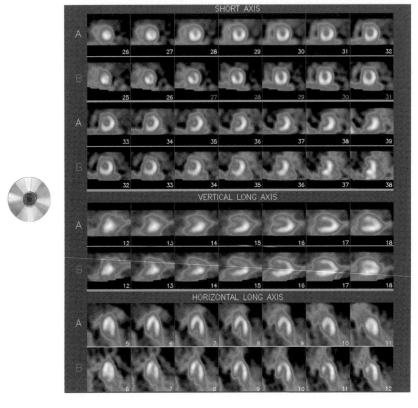

**Fig. 14-43.** Same images as in Fig. 14-42 in color.

**Fig. 14-44.** (*Top right*) Quantification of the SPECT slices in Figs. 14-42 and 14-43. A small anterolateral defect is present on the apical, midventricular, and basal slices. Some minor defect reversibility is quantitatively present.

**Fig. 14-45.** (*Bottom right*) Gated-SPECT movie of the slices shown in Figs. 14-42 and 14-43. Regional wall motion and thickening is normal in the area of the apparent defect.

| Perfusion Defect Size (%LV) | | | | | |
|---|---|---|---|---|---|
| | Apical | MVent | Basal | Apex | Total |
| A | 0 | 2 | 2 | 0 | 4 |
| B | 2 | 0 | 0 | 0 | 2 |
| Dif | 2 | -2 | -2 | 0 | -2 |
| % | 100 % | -100 % | -100 % | 0 % | -50 % |

— Normal
— A, STRESS
— B, REST
Data Base: MIBI

APICAL
Min_A= 65%  Ext_A=31%
Min_B  59%  Ext_B=34%

MID-VENTRICLE
Min_A= 62%  Ext_A=18%
Min_B  62%  Ext_B= 0%

BASAL
Min_A= 63%  Ext_A=41%
Min_B  61%  Ext_B=23%

APEX
Min_A= 89%  Ext_A= 0%
Min_B= 84%  Ext_B= 0%

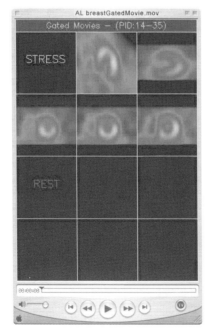

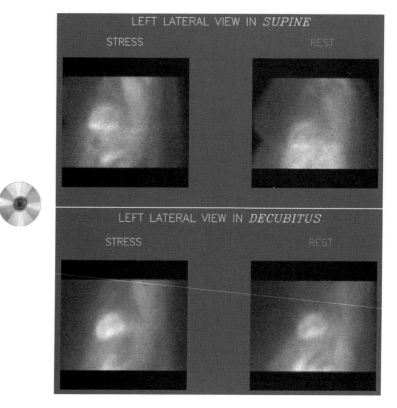

**Fig. 14-46.** Planar supine and right-side decubitus left lateral images of the same patient as in Fig. 14-41 to 14-45. The right-side decubitus images are normal because in this position the breast moves to the middle of the chest. The supine images, the position in which the SPECT images were acquired, show attenuation of the anterior wall by breast tissue. The constellation of findings on the rotating images, these planar images and gated-SPECT movie, suggest that breast attenuation may be responsible for the anterior defect. This patient had normal coronary arteries on coronary angiography.

## BREAST ATTENUATION

*Recognition*
Shadow on rotating images.
Normal regional wall motion on gated SPECT.
*Preventive measure*
None.
*Corrective measure*
Attenuation correction.

## Noncardiac Radiotracer Uptake (Fig. 14-47 to Fig. 14-52)

The rotating images should not only be analyzed for motion and attenuation, but also for other noncardiac radiotracer uptake that may be of significance for the interpretation of the study. One should routinely watch for noncardiac uptake in the axilla, mediastinum, breasts, lungs, and elsewhere as such uptake may represent malignancies.

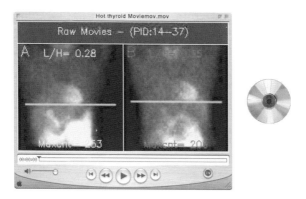

**Fig. 14-47.** On these rotating planar projection images one can note at the top of the field of view radiotracer uptake in the thyroid gland. This is most likely due to suboptimal labeling of the radiopharmaceutical. Free Tc-99m-pertechnetate accumulates in thyroid gland and mucosa of the stomach.

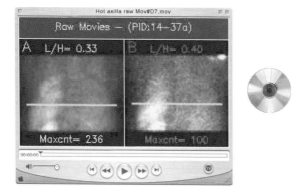

**Fig. 14-48.** The rotating planar projection image on the rest study show intense radiotracer uptake in the right axilla. One should attempt to understand the cause for such a finding. This is important, as radiotracer uptake in the axilla could indicate malignancy in an axillary lymph node. The uptake is then usually present on both the stress and rest images. The intensity of uptake and presence in the rest study only suggest that contamination of skin or gown with radiotracer is a more likely cause. One should try to clarify this finding by discussion with the nuclear medicine technologist.

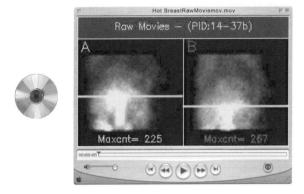

**Fig. 14-49.** On the rotating images abnormal radiotracer uptake can be noted in both breasts. This is always an abnormal finding that should be reported. It is feasible that the woman is lactating, has a bilateral infection, or may have a malignancy.

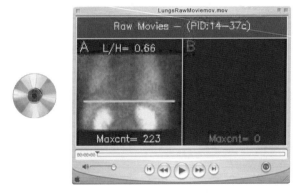

**Fig. 14-50.** The rotating stress images show markedly increased pulmonary uptake of radiotracer. This image pattern, seen in conjunction with a reversible myocardial perfusion abnormality, may be a marker of transient ischemic left ventricular dysfunction and is a predictor a poor outcome. On the images the heart is clearly enlarged and this patient may have chronic congestive heart failure.

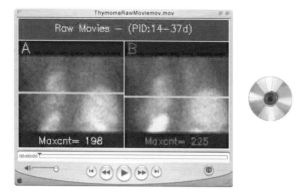

**Fig. 14-51.** The rotating planar projection images show clearly abnormal radiotracer uptake to the right side of the heart. This abnormal finding was mentioned in the report. The patient was later found to have a thymoma.

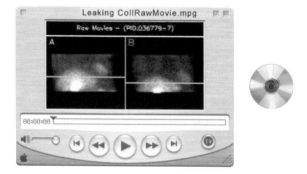

**Fig. 14-52.** Rotating stress (**A**) and rest (**B**) planar projection images. During the rotation of the stress images a bright "glow" appears on the top of the images in the anterior positions. This is most likely due to "leaking" radioactivity from outside the field of view between the mounted collimator and the gamma camera detector head. The technologist must investigate the cause of this artifact by surveying the patient's gown, neck, and arms for contamination or extravasation of injected dose. It is also possible that the collimator is not mounted correctly on the camera head. This is potentially dangerous because the collimator could fall off and injure the patient. If the collimator is mounted correctly, one can purchase lead guards that cover the slit between the collimator and camera and will prevent this artifact from recurring.

## *Reconstructed Tomographic Slices*
## *Correct Orientation of Tomographic Axis*
## *and Alignment of Slices (Fig. 14-53 to Fig. 14-56)*

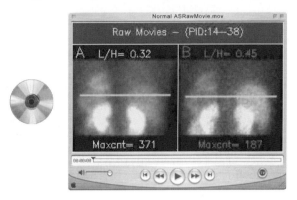

**Fig. 14-53.** Cine display of rotating planar projection images. The images were acquired using a circular orbit and 360° arc. In this, and all other movies of projection images, the stress study is on the left and the rest study on the right. The horizontal white line serves as a reference mark and is placed by the technologist at approximately the level of the left ventricular apex. The most convenient display speed for inspecting these images is at 10 frames/second. The lung/heart ratio (L/H) is displayed, as is the maximal count density/pixel within the left ventricle. The lung/heart ratio is normal on the stress images (0.32) and upper limit of normal on the rest images (0.45). The count density in the left ventricle on the stress images is excellent (371/pixel) and adequate on the rest images (187/pixel). There is no significant patient motion. No breast shadow is noted. The liver has cleared most of the radiotracer on the stress images into the gallbladder and gastrointestinal tract. On the rest images moderate residual radiotracer activity is still present in the liver. The gall bladder is prominent. On the stress and rest images both kidneys can be seen on the posterior projections of the 360° acquisition.

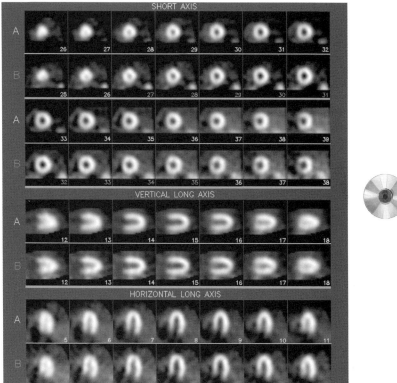

**Fig. 14-54.** Reconstructed SPECT slices of the raw projection data shown in Fig. 14-53. The display of reconstructed slices in this and other images adheres to ACC/AHA/ASNC/SNM standards for display of tomographic images. The short-axis (SA) slices are displayed on top, the vertical long-axis (VLA) slices in the middle and the horizontal long-axis (HLA) slices on the bottom. The rows marked with "A" show the stress images and rows marked with "B" show rest images. The SA slices are displayed from apex (#26 and # 25) to base (#39 and # 38); the VLA slices are displayed from septum (#12) to lateral wall (#18); the HLA are displayed from inferior wall (#5 and #6) to anterior wall (#11 and #12). This is an example of normal SPECT images.

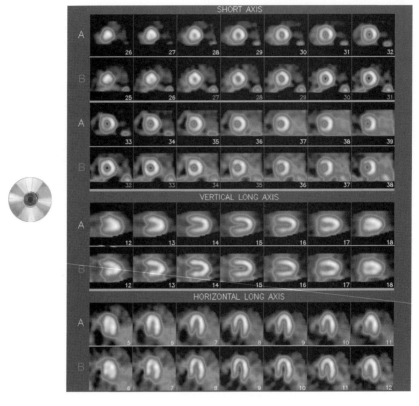

**Fig. 14-55.** Same images as in Fig. 14-54 in color.

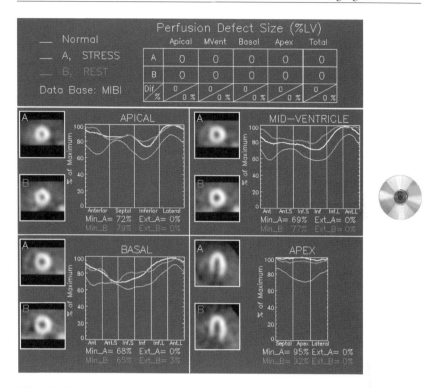

**Fig. 14-56.** Quantification of the SPECT slices in Figs. 14-54 and 14-55 using circumferential count distribution profile analysis. The yellow curves represent the count distribution on the stress images and the red curves represent the rest images. The white curve represents the lower limit of normal radiotracer distribution (mean minus two standard deviations). The stress and rest curves are within the lower limit of normal in the apical, midventricular, and basal short-axis slices. The apical segment is quantified from a mid horizontal long-axis slice and is normal as well. In the table at the top the results of computer quantification are shown. No defects are quantified. These are quantitatively normal SPECT images.

## INCORRECT ORIENTATION OF TOMOGRAPHIC AXIS (FIG. 14-57 TO FIG. 14-60)

The first step in reconstruction of tomographic images is to create tomographic slices that are oriented along the anatomical axis of the body, resulting in transverse, coronal and sagittal slices. Since the heart is positioned in the chest at an angle to the body axis, interpretation of

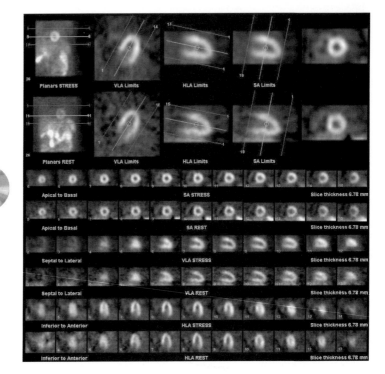

**Fig. 14-57.** Correct slicing. In order obtain tomographic slices of the heart perpendicular to the anatomic axis of the left ventricular limits of slicing (red lines) and direction of long axis (green lines) must be chosen on transverse and sagital body slices. Correct limits of slicing ensure that tomographic slices of the entire heart are obtained. Most important for the generation of cardiac slices that meet standards of tomographic display is the selection of the anatomic axis of the left ventricle by the technologist. The figure shows correct selection of the angles of slicing and of limits of slicing. This results in SPECT images of the heart that meet standards of display. Short-axis slices should be circular with the right ventricle at the same level as the left. The vertical long-axis images should show a horseshoe with the closed tip pointing to the right. The anterior and inferior wall should be of approximately equal length. The inferior wall should be parallel to the lower border of the image. The horizontal long-axis image should show a horseshoe configuration with the closed tip pointing upward. The right ventricle is to the left. The septum in the middle should be one-half to three-quarters of the lateral wall. This is achieved by correct selection of angles of slicing.

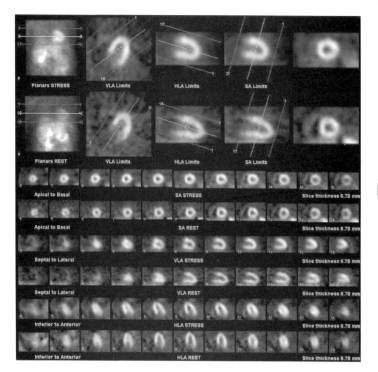

**Fig. 14-58.** Incorrect slicing (vertical). In this example the angle of the anatomical long axis of the left ventricle as a direction for slicing is incorrectly selected for the stress vertical long-axis limits. The angles for the rest images are correct. The incorrect angles result in nonstandard stress slices of the left ventricle. This is best appreciated in the horizontal long-axis slices. The stress images are at an unusual angle and point to the left. The stress vertical long-axis slices are apparently foreshortened compared to the rest slices. Some of the short-axis slices have an elliptical rather than circular shape.

conventional coronal, transverse, and sagittal slices is difficult because the walls of the heart are cut tangentially. Therefore, tomographic cuts through the heart must be reoriented according to the anatomical axis of the *left ventricle*. Two conceivable mistakes can be made: (1) The selection of long axis is not precisely along the anatomical axis of the heart. (2) The orientation of the selected axis in the stress and rest images

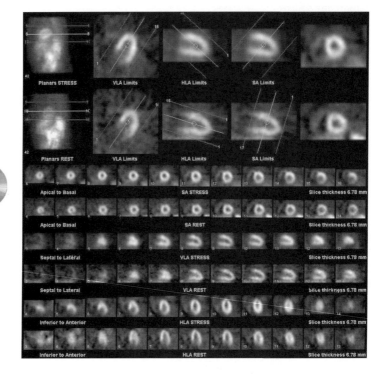

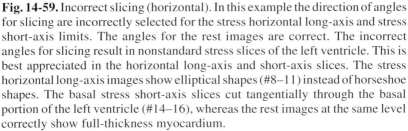

**Fig. 14-59.** Incorrect slicing (horizontal). In this example the direction of angles for slicing are incorrectly selected for the stress horizontal long-axis and stress short-axis limits. The angles for the rest images are correct. The incorrect angles for slicing result in nonstandard stress slices of the left ventricle. This is best appreciated in the horizontal long-axis and short-axis slices. The stress horizontal long-axis images show elliptical shapes (#8–11) instead of horseshoe shapes. The basal stress short-axis slices cut tangentially through the basal portion of the left ventricle (#14–16), whereas the rest images at the same level correctly show full-thickness myocardium.

are not parallel. These errors can be recognized relatively easily, because the slices "do not look" like usual images. Although the eye usually may be able to deal with slight deviations in slicing, quantification of images and inspection of bull's eye display alone can lead to incorrect conclusions.

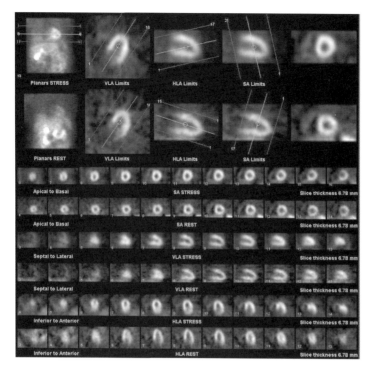

**Fig. 14-60.** Incorrect slicing (short axis). In this example the angles for direction for slicing are incorrectly selected for the stress horizontal long-axis and stress short-axis limits. The angles for the rest images are correct. The incorrect angles for slicing result in nonstandard stress slices of the left ventricle. This is best appreciated in the horizontal long-axis and short-axis slices. The stress horizontal long axis images show elliptical shapes (#7–9) instead of horseshoe shapes. The basal stress short axis slices cut tangentially through the anteroseptal basal portion of the left ventricle (#14–16), whereas the rest images at the same level still show full-thickness myocardium.

## INCORRECT AXIS ORIENTATION

*Recognition*

Inspection of anatomical appearance of reconstructed slices.

Compare anatomical appearance of slices in stress and rest studies.

*Preventive measure*

Appropriate training of technologist with understanding of anatomy and technology.

*Corrective measure*

Repeat processing with correct axis selection.

## MISALIGNMENT OF SLICES ON DISPLAY (FIG. 14-61 TO FIG. 14-65)

Interpretation of stress–rest SPECT slices consists of comparison of myocardial perfusion patterns in stress and rest reconstructed slices. In order for comparison to be valid, slices must be well aligned, i.e., apical and basal slice selections must match. Misalignment in display may lead

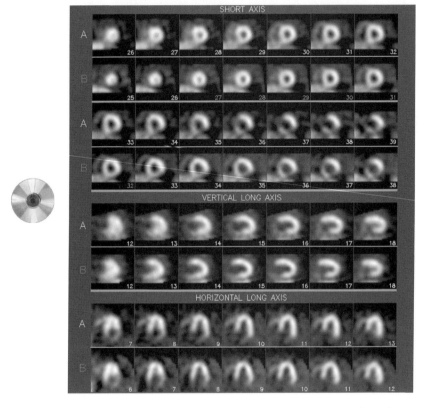

**Fig. 14-61.** The tomographic slices of this SPECT study were not aligned correctly. All stress slices should be moved one position to the right in order to match the rest study. This patient has a relatively small fixed inferolateral basal defect, as can be appreciated in the vertical and horizontal long-axis slices. Because of the misalignment of slices, one could erroneously conclude that the defect is partially reversible.

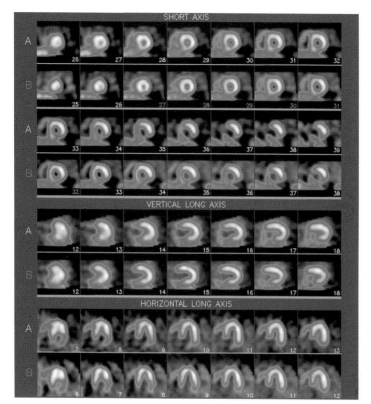

**Fig. 14-62.** Same images as in Fig. 14-61 in color.

to misinterpretations, e.g., erroneous transient ventricular dilation or erroneous defect reversibility. Mistakes can be avoided by careful inspection of the arrangement of reconstructed stress and rest slices on display, e.g., the first apical slices showing left ventricular cavity and

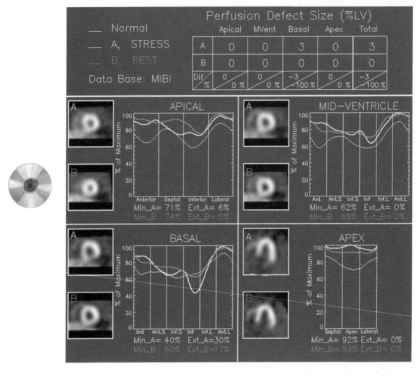

**Fig. 14-63.** Quantification of the stress and rest SPECT slices in Figs. 14-61 and 14-62. Because of misalignment quantification shows a small reversible inferolateral basal defect.

first slice showing membranous septum should be well aligned. Nevertheless, it may not always be possible to align images; in markedly abnormal studies with true transient dilation of the left ventricle, it may not be possible to make a match.

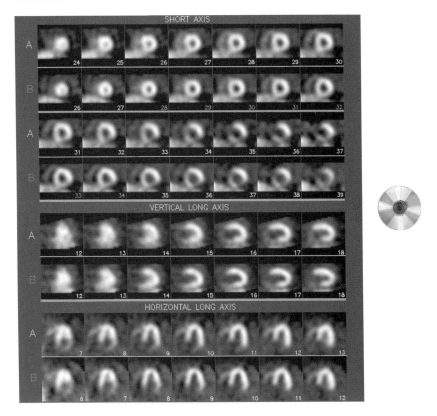

**Fig. 14-64.** Same SPECT study as in Figs. 14-61 and 14-62 with correct alignment. The inferolateral basal defect appears fixed.

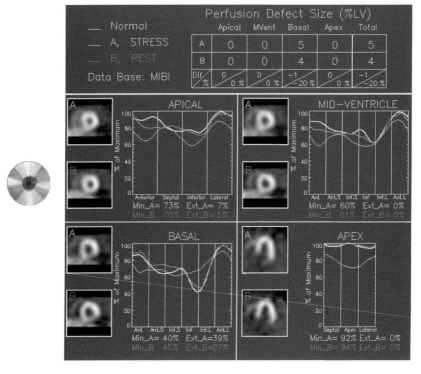

**Fig. 14-65.** Quantification of the stress and rest SPECT slices in Fig. 14-48. Because of correct alignment quantification shows a small fixed inferolateral basal defect (5% of left ventricle).

## MISALIGNMENT

*Recognition*

Careful inspection of match at apex and base of reconstructed stress and rest slices.

*Preventive measure*

Appropriate training of technologist.

The written procedure protocol should provide instruction on how to align images.

*Corrective measure*

Repeat processing with correct comparative display of slices.

## INTENSE GASTROINTESTINAL UPTAKE (FIG. 14-66 TO FIG. 14-73)

Using Tc-99m-labeled agents, intense gastrointestinal uptake of radiopharmaceuticals can be a serious problem, generally after pharmacological stress and on resting images. This is particularly true if "hot" extracardiac activity is present immediately adjacent to the heart, i.e., the inferior wall. Intense uptake at a distance from the heart, i.e., gallbladder and lower intestines usually do not cause many problems. That is, unless a very hot organ is present within the selected block for backprojection and reconstruction. This may results in the so-called "northern light" artifact.

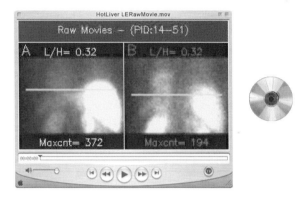

**Fig. 14-66.** Adenosine stress and rest rotating projection images of a female patient. During adenosine infusion, the patient was supine on the imaging table. One can appreciate intense radiotracer uptake in the liver. Technical problems during filtered backprojection may be anticipated.

Measures to reduce the amount gastrointestinal activity are inconsistently effective. Low level of exercise may decrease splanchnic uptake. Drinking a large amount of fluid may help to move radioactivity through the gastrointestinal tract.

Intense gastrointestinal activity immediately adjacent to the heart may cause interpretive problems in several ways:

1. Superimposition of activity on the inferior left ventricular wall, making analysis of inferior wall impossible.
2. Scattering of photons into the left ventricular inferior wall: a fixed inferior defect may appear reversible.
3. Back projection and filtering artifact resulting in erroneous defects (6).

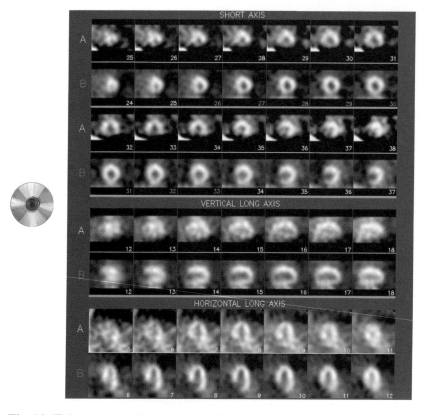

**Fig. 14-67.** Reconstructed tomographic slices of the images in Fig. 14-66. The rest images are of acceptable quality. However, the stress images are of suboptimal quality with substantial background noise. There is an inferior wall defect on the stress images that is not present at rest. Because of intense liver uptake adjacent to the heart, one should be concerned about a filtered backprojection artifact. It is conceivable that the filter-suppressed image data in the inferior wall of the heart in the presence of the hot liver.

**Fig. 14-68.** Same images as in Fig. 14-67 in color.

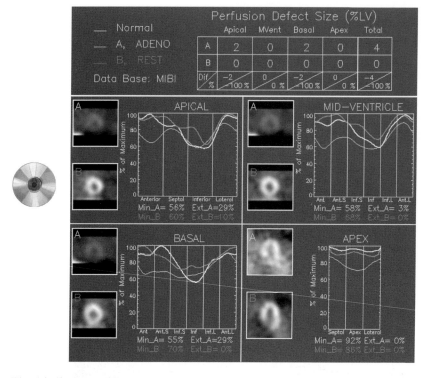

| | Perfusion Defect Size (%LV) | | | | |
| --- | --- | --- | --- | --- | --- |
| —— Normal | Apical | MVent | Basal | Apex | Total |
| —— A, ADENO | A | 2 | 0 | 2 | 0 | 4 |
| —— B, REST | B | 0 | 0 | 0 | 0 | 0 |
| Data Base: MIBI | Dif % | -2 / -100% | 0 / 0% | -2 / -100% | 0 / 0% | -4 / -100% |

APICAL — Min_A= 56% Ext_A=29% / Min_B 60% Ext_B=10%

MID—VENTRICLE — Min_A= 58% Ext_A= 3% / Min_B 68% Ext_B= 0%

BASAL — Min_A= 55% Ext_A=29% / Min_B 70% Ext_B= 0%

APEX — Min_A= 92% Ext_A= 0% / Min_B= 86% Ext_B= 0%

**Fig. 14-69.** Quantification of the images in Figs. 14-67 and 14-68. The circumferential profiles show an inferior defect that is reversible at rest. Because of intense adjacent liver uptake, one should be concerned about the possibility of a filtered backprojection artifact. It is conceivable that the filter suppressed image data in the inferior wall of the heart in the presence of the hot liver.

**Fig. 14-70.** (*Top right*) Rotating projection images of the same patient as in Figs. 14-66–14-69. Since the first study was considered potentially artifactual, adenosine stress test was repeated with simultaneous low-level (Bruce 1) treadmill exercise. On the repeat stress images, liver uptake is markedly less compared to that in Fig. 14-66.

**Fig. 14-71.** (*Bottom right*) Reconstructed tomographic slices of the images in Fig. 14-70. The stress images are of much better quality than those in Fig. 14-67. A small inferior myocardial perfusion defect is present after stress and at rest.

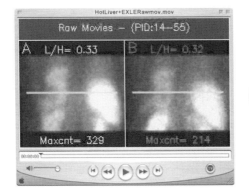

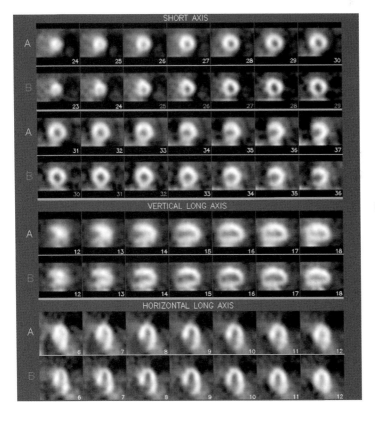

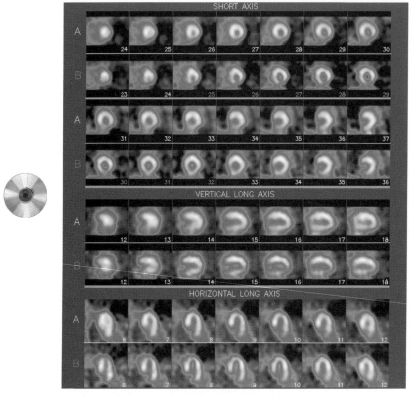

**Fig. 14-72.** Same images as in Fig. 14-71 in color.

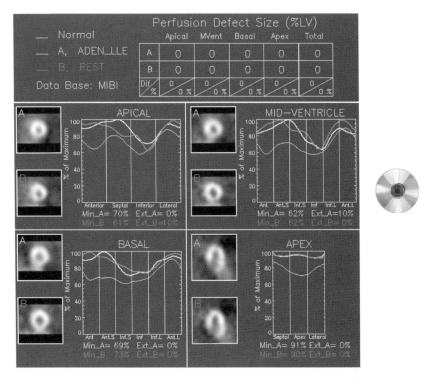

**Fig. 14-73.** Quantification of the images in Figs. 14-71 and 14-72. The small inferior defect is not quantifiable against the Sestamibi normal database and probably due to inferior attenuation.

## GASTROINTESTINAL UPTAKE

> *Recognition*
> Obvious on rotating images and reconstructed slices.
> *Preventive measure*
> Ingestion of large amount of fluid before imaging (inconsistent result).
> Low level exercise during injection of radiopharmaceutical.
> *Corrective measure*
> Wait until radioactivity has moved down the intestinal tract and repeat imaging
> Ingestion of large amount of fluid.

QUANTIFICATION ERRORS (FIG. 14-74 TO FIG. 14-82)

Image quantification may be a great help for consistency in interpretation. However, when used in an uncritical way, it may lead to errors. It is important that visual analysis of reconstructed slices and image quantification are considered together. Information from visual and

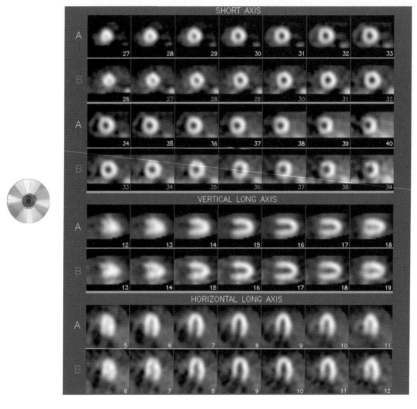

**Fig. 14-74.** Errors can be made in the process of image quantification. In this normal SPECT study (also shown as Fig. 14-54) the technologist erroneously selected too many basal slices. Slices selected for quantification are indicated in color. Of the stress study, slices #28–#40, and of the rest study, slices #27–#39, were included for quantification. It can be appreciated that the membranous septum is present in the last two basal slices.

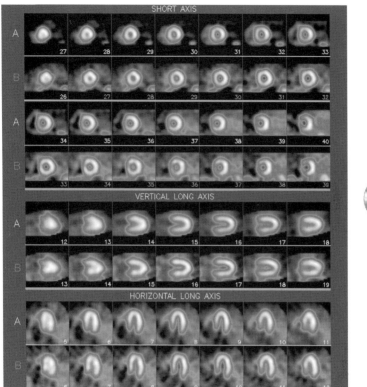

**Fig. 14-75.** Same images as in figure 15-74 in color.

quantitative analysis should be concordant. Inappropriate selection of slices may result in discordant quantification. For instance, inclusion of too many basal slices (of a normal study) may result in quantification of an erroneous septal defect, whereas inclusion of too few basal slices (e.g., of a study with a septal defect), may result in an erroneously normal study by quantification.

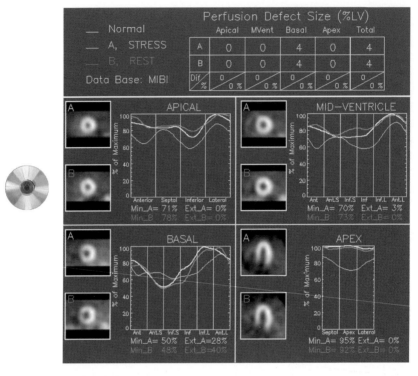

**Fig. 14-76.** Quantification of the tomographic images in Figs. 14-74 and 14-75. Because of the inclusion of too many basal slices, a small fixed basal septal defect is quantified. This is an error and represents the membranous septum. Correct quantification of these images is shown in Fig. 14-56.

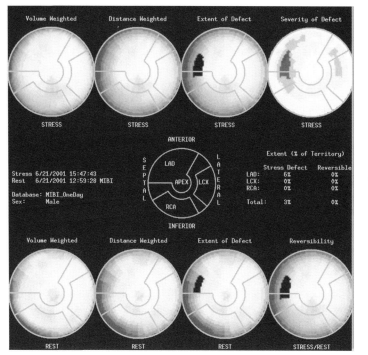

**Fig. 14-77.** Bull's eye display of the same reconstruction error as in Fig. 14-76. An erroneous septal defect (6%) is present in the LAD territory.

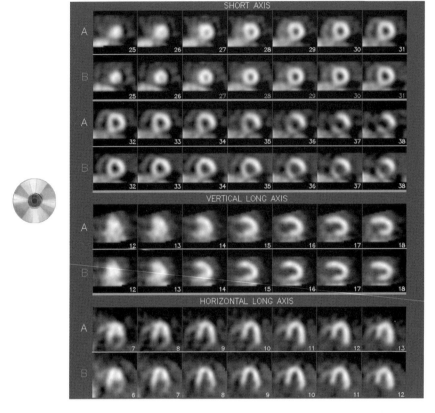

**Fig. 14-78.** Reconstructed SPECT images with a fixed inferolateral basal myocardial perfusion defect (slices #34–36). Note also that the inferior wall is shorter than the anterior wall (indicating basal inferior defect) on the vertical long axis slices. The technologist, attempting not to include the membranous septum, included too few basal slices. Slices selected for quantification are indicated in color. Only slices #27–#31 were included for quantification. It can be appreciated that the basal defect is not included.

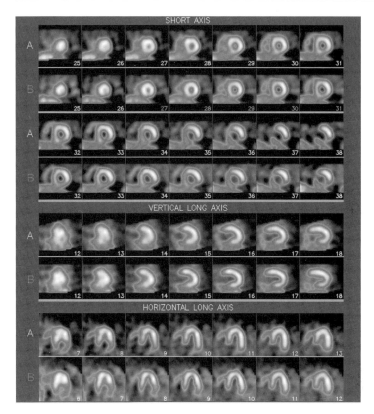

**Fig. 14-79.** Same images as in Fig. 14-78 in color.

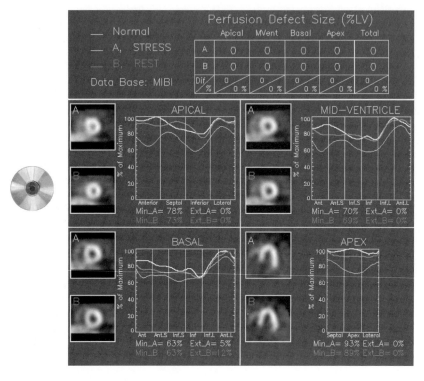

**Fig. 14-80.** Quantification of tomographic images in Figs. 14-78 and 14-79. Because of the inclusion of too few slices, the basal defect is not quantified and quantitatively the study is normal.

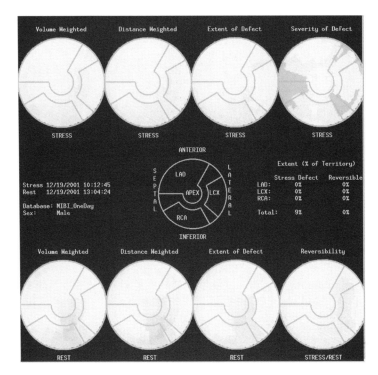

**Fig. 14-81.** Bull's eye display of the same reconstruction error as in Fig. 14-80. No defect is displayed.

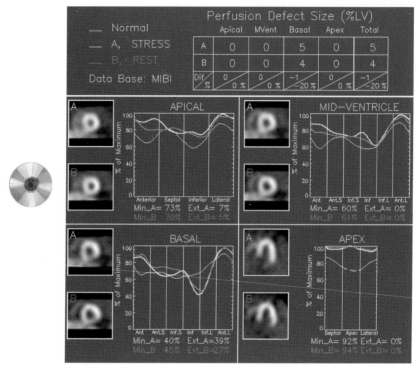

**Fig. 14-82.** Correct quantification of tomographic images in Figs. 14-78 and 14-79. A small fixed inferolateral basal defect is quantified.

## QUANTIFICATION ERRORS

---

*Recognition*
Integrate visual interpretation of images with results of quantification.
*Preventive measure*
Understand limitations of quantitative program.
*Corrective measure*
Repeat processing and quantification.
Integrate other clinical and imaging information in final interpretation.

---

### FILTERING (FIG. 14-83 TO FIG. 14-88)

Filtering is applied to remove noise from the images and "make them look better." The low-pass Butterworth filter is currently considered standard for cardiac SPECT imaging. Of the two variables of this filter, "order and cut-off," only the Nyquist frequency cut-off is to be considered.

No true standardization exists for filter settings, only general guidelines. There is no standardization of the effect of a given filter cut-off value using filters provided by different vendors. It is recommended that one check with the vendor for preferred cut-off values. Furthermore, images with different imaging characteristics require different filter cut-offs. For example, images acquired using different imaging protocols, images acquired with high dose or low dose, images with significant or little extra cardiac activity, each may need a different filter cut-off.

Nevertheless, using the equipment available in an imaging facility, one should develop *standard filter settings* for images acquired with routinely used protocols in order to achieve reproducible image quality.

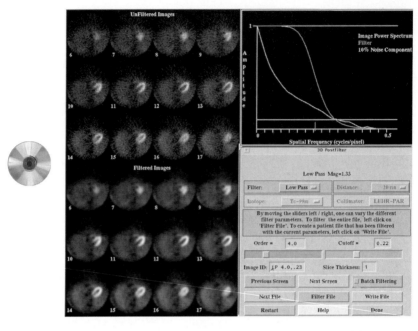

**Fig. 14-83.** Inconsistent or incorrect use of filters may impact significantly on image quality. The figure in the left panel shows unfiltered transverse axis SPECT images (top) and filtered images (bottom). A low-pass Butterworth filter is used. The right panel shows the image power spectrum (green curve), which is characteristic for an individual image. High frequencies generally represent "noise," whereas low frequencies represent "signal" and presumably true image components. The filter (orange curve) is characterized by order, i.e., slope of the curve, and most importantly by the cutoff. The selection of the cutoff level determines how much noise is suppressed and how smooth or blurred the filtered image will look. The filter used for these images is standard in our laboratory and has an order of 4.0 and cutoff of 0.22.

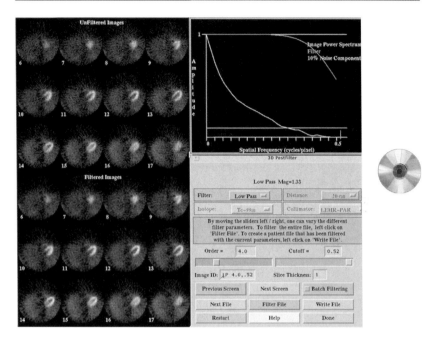

**Fig. 14-84.** The filter used for the images in the left panel (bottom) has an order of 4.0 and cutoff of 0.52. The orange curve is moved to the far right. Basically all noise is left in the images by the filter. The unfiltered and filtered images look similar in quality.

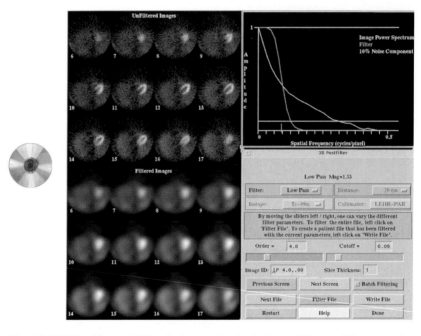

**Fig. 14-85.** The filter used for the images in the left panel (bottom) has an order of 4.0 and cutoff of 0.09. The orange curve is moved to the far left. The filter has suppressed all noise. The filtered images are extremely blurred with loss of image detail.

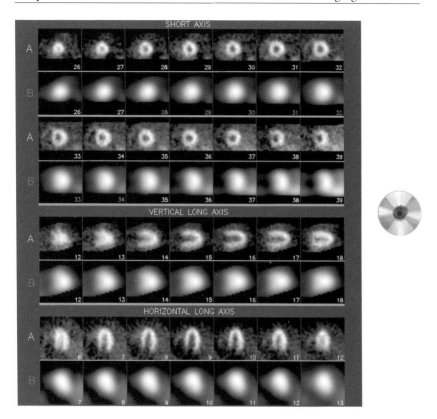

**Fig. 14-86.** Reconstructed tomographic slices of the normal SPECT study shown in Fig. 14-39. The images in rows "A" were filtered with a high cutoff value (0.52), whereas the images in rows "B" were filtered with a low cutoff value (0.09). The results of using the appropriate filter cutoff (0.22) are shown in Fig. 14-39.

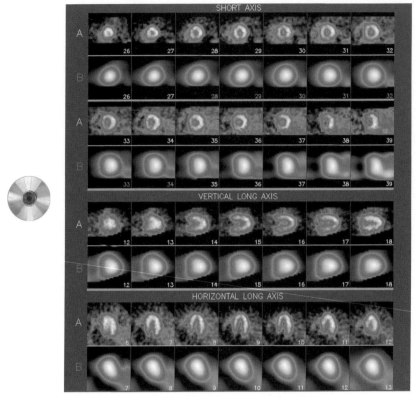

**Fig. 14-87.** Same images as in Fig. 14-86 in color.

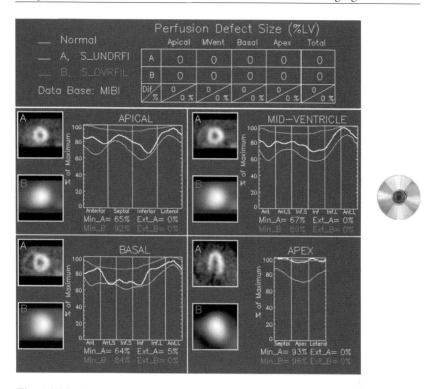

**Fig. 14-88.** Quantification of the tomographic slices in Fig. 14-86. The circumferential profile of the heavily smoothed images is smooth and almost a straight line. The circumferential count profile of the underfiltered images shows considerably greater noise and approaches in some segments the lower limit of normal. Although both curves of this example are within the normal range, one can appreciate that circumferential count profiles of low-count and unfiltered images fall outside the normal reference range due to "noise" and create false-positive defects.

## FILTERING ERRORS

*Recognition*
Inspection of reconstructed slices.
Images should not be exceedingly blurred or noisy.
*Preventive measure*
Appropriate training of technologist.
Written procedure protocol with standard filter selection.
*Corrective measure*
Repeat processing of slices with appropriate filter selection.

## SYNCHRONIZATION ERROR ECG-GATED SPECT
## (FIG. 14-89 TO FIG. 14-95)

The validity of information gained from ECG-gated SPECT depends on a regular heart rate and appropriate synchronization with the ECG. This is a much-ignored aspect of QC of gated SPECT imaging.

The occurrence of irregular heart rate results in missed data during image acquisition and may lead to errors in calculation of ejection fraction and display of cardiac function. Theoretically, a gated SPECT study acquired with 8 frames per cardiac cycle is more likely to be corrupted by arrhythmias than a study acquired with 16 frames per cycle.

ECG gating error may be suspected from the inspection of the rotating planar projection images. If an arrhythmia occurred at a certain time point during SPECT acquisition, one or more planar projection images may contain fewer total counts than the other may. This may result in "flashing" (darker images) during the movie display. This can also be displayed graphically (7).

ECG gating error may also be suspected from movie display of reconstructed slices. Normally there is a gradual change in color from systole (brightest color) to diastole (darkest color). If significant irregular heart

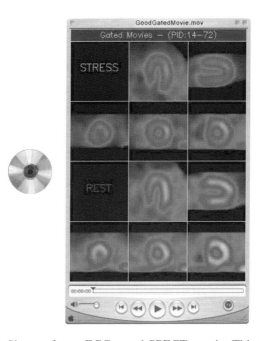

**Fig. 14-89.** Sixteen-frame ECG-gated SPECT movie. This is a good quality study. There is gradual change in color from diastole to systole (blue to white). Regional wall motion and wall thickening are normal.

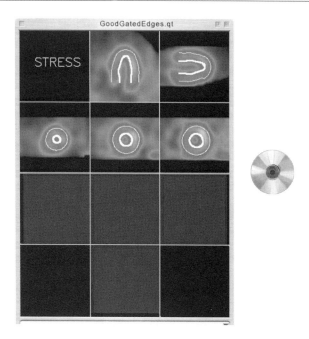

**Fig. 14-90.** ECG-gated SPECT movie. Display of computer-derived endocardial edges for calculation of left ventricular ejection fraction of gated SPECT movie shown in Fig. 14-89.

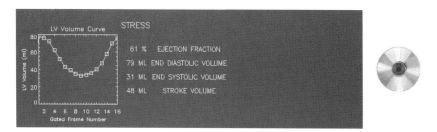

**Fig. 14-91.** Sixteen-frame left ventricular (LV) volume curve of Figs. 14-89 and 14-90. The left ventricular volume curve is derived from the sum of volumes determined on the basis of number of voxels within the endocardial boundaries of each individual short-axis slice and the apical cap. The volume curve shows a physiologic shape and thus credible ejection fraction. End diastolic and end systolic volumes are shown as well.

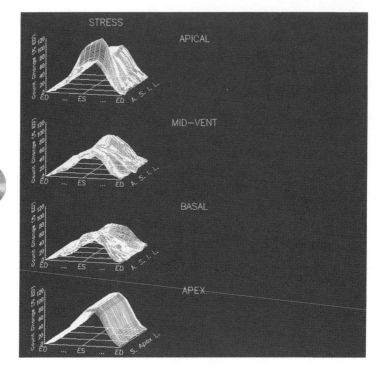
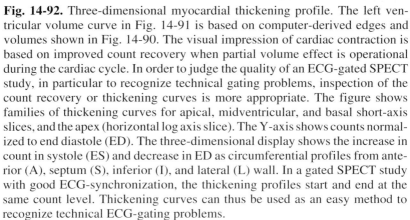

**Fig. 14-92.** Three-dimensional myocardial thickening profile. The left ventricular volume curve in Fig. 14-91 is based on computer-derived edges and
volumes shown in Fig. 14-90. The visual impression of cardiac contraction is
based on improved count recovery when partial volume effect is operational
during the cardiac cycle. In order to judge the quality of an ECG-gated SPECT
study, in particular to recognize technical gating problems, inspection of the
count recovery or thickening curves is more appropriate. The figure shows
families of thickening curves for apical, midventricular, and basal short-axis
slices, and the apex (horizontal log axis slice). The Y-axis shows counts normalized to end diastole (ED). The three-dimensional display shows the increase in
count in systole (ES) and decrease in ED as circumferential profiles from anterior (A), septum (S), inferior (I), and lateral (L) wall. In a gated SPECT study
with good ECG-synchronization, the thickening profiles start and end at the
same count level. Thickening curves can thus be used as an easy method to
recognize technical ECG-gating problems.

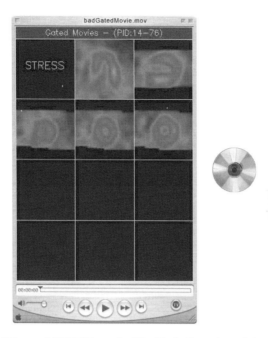

**Fig. 14-93.** ECG-gated SPECT movie. The "jerky" motion of the movie should raise the suspicion of a technical ECG-gating problem. There appears to be an abrupt transition at end diastole.

rate occurred, the end diastolic frame is abruptly darker than the preceding frames.

One can also inspect the morphology of the left volume curve. The volume curve should start and end at approximately the same end diastolic volume and display a well-defined systolic nadir. When heart rate during acquisition is significantly irregular, the volume curve is distorted.

Since the visual appearance of motion and contraction on gated SPECT is due to the greater count recovery during cardiac contraction because of the partial volume effect, it is more appropriate to inspect myocardial-thickening curves (8). In the absence of arrhythmias, myocardial counts at both ends of the thickening curve, end diastole, are the similar. In case of irregular heart rate, counts at the end of the thickening curve are lower than those at the beginning of the curve.

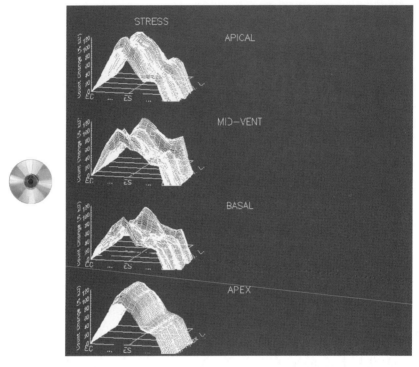

**Fig. 14-94.** Three-dimensional myocardial thickening profile of the gated SPECT study shown in Fig. 14-93. In contrast to the thickening profiles shown in Fig. 14-92, the counts in end diastole (ED) at the end of the cardiac cycle fall below count values in ED at the beginning of the cardiac cycle. This is due to heart rate variability and may invalidate calculation of ejection fraction. Quality control for ECG-gating problems is often ignored.

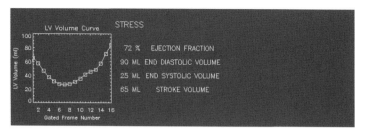

**Fig. 14-95.** Sixteen-frame left ventricular (LV) volume curve of the ECG-gated SPECT study shown in Figs. 14-93 and 14-94. The volume curve does not have a "physiological appearance." It is uncertain which of the two points for end diastole should be used for calculation of ejection fraction. The validity of the calculation of ejection fraction can be questioned. Note: In contrast to Fig. 14-91 where end diastolic counts in frame #1 are similar to those in frame #16, in this geometrically derived curve end diastolic volume in frame #16 is larger than that in frame #1.

## ECG GATING PROBLEMS

> *Recognition*
> Flashing on display of rotating planar projection images.
> Flashing on display of gated SPECT movie.
> Curve displaying in each frame of projection images.
> LV volume curve.
> Thickening curve.
> *Preventive measure*
> Do not acquire ECG-gated SPECT in patients with irregular heart rate.
> *Corrective measure*
> None.

## *Planar Myocardial Perfusion Imaging (Fig. 14-96 to Fig. 14-98)*

### BREAST ATTENUATION

Breast attenuation is a serious problem with planar myocardial perfusion imaging. This is in marked contrast to SPECT imaging. In planar imaging only three projection images are acquired. Breast attenuation defects may make images that are affected uninterpretable; thus, interpretation is then limited to the one or two remaining images, thereby seriously limiting the diagnostic yield of planar myocardial perfusion imaging *(2)*.

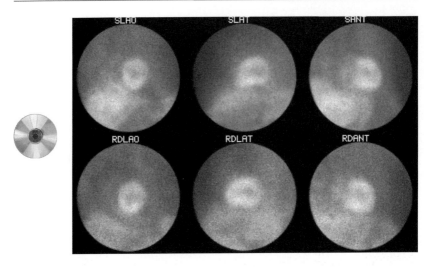

**Fig. 14-96.** Planar adenosine stress (S)–redistribution (RD) thallium-201 images of a patient with large breasts. There appears to be a reversible anterior wall defect on the left anterior oblique (LAO) and left lateral (LAT) images and anterior images (ANT). However, there are also a large breast shadow visible, in particular, on the LAO and ANT images. This could be a cause for anterior defects. Because the LAT images are acquired in right-side decubitus position, breast attenuation is usually not a problem on these views. In order to interpret these images, the overlap of breast over the heart should be defined.

The only planar image not likely to be affected by breast attenuation is the left lateral right-side decubitus image. With the patient lying on the right side, the left breast moves away from the heart and the anterior wall and inferior wall can be imaged without attenuation.

We have found that breast markers (small plastic tubing filled with radioisotope) that outline the contours of the breast are useful for recognizing breast attenuation *(2)*. However, although one may identify the presence of breast attenuation, one cannot exclude the presence of an ischemic myocardial perfusion defect as well.

In many laboratories planar imaging is currently only performed in overweight patients who are too heavy for SPECT imaging tables. In these obese patients, it is our policy to be conservative in interpreting planar images in the obese. Only *unequivocally* abnormal features are reported as abnormal. More subtle inhomogeneities are presumed to be equivocal or due to attenuation.

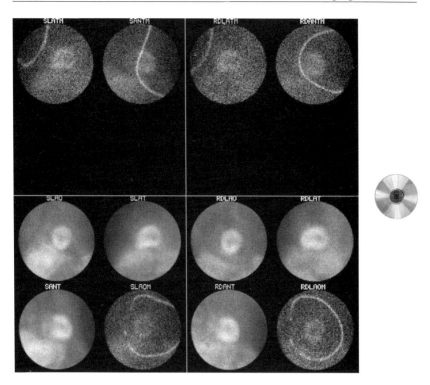

**Fig. 14-97.** Same thallium-201 images as in Fig. 14-96. In addition, there are images with radioactive line sources to mark the contours of the breast. The breast markers in the LAO views show that the left breast is indeed large and completely covers the entire heart in this projection. This will generally result in homogeneous attenuation and not in regional defects. The contour of the breast in the ANT view is across the base of the heart and does not match up with the mild anteroapical perfusion defect in this view. The breast markers in the LAT view confirm that the breast is not overlying the heart. Knowing the exact location of the contours of the breast relative to the heart and the observed perfusion defects is helpful in concluding that this patients most likely has a true anteroapical and lateral reversible myocardial perfusion defect.

## PLANAR IMAGING: BREAST ATTENUATION

> *Recognition*
> Planar images with breast markers.
> *Preventive measure*
> None.
> *Corrective measure*
> None.

### INFERIOR ATTENUATION

As discussed under SPECT imaging, inferior attenuation is importantly dependent on imaging position. Steep 60° left-anterior-oblique and 90° left-lateral-planar images with patient in supine position during image acquisition have high likelihood of inferior attenuation artifacts. However, a left-lateral-planar image acquired with the patient in right-side decubitus is not affected by inferior attenuation *(1)*.

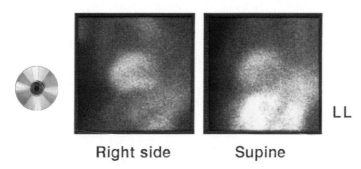

**Right side          Supine**

**Fig. 14-98.** Inferior attenuation by the left hemi-diaphragm occurs in about 25% of patients when imaging is performed in supine position. Diaphragmatic attenuation can be demonstrated by comparing two planar left lateral (LL) images, one supine and another one with the patient in right-side decubitus position. The figure shows an example of inferior attenuation. The supine LL image (right) shows an apparent inferobasal myocardial perfusion defect. This defect is not present on a second LL image (left) taken a few minutes later with the patient in right-side decubitus position. The latter image is normal. Therefore, there is attenuation when the patient is supine.

### PLANAR IMAGING INSUSION ATTENUATION

> *Recognition*
> Inferior defect on supine steep left anterior oblique or left lateral planar images.
> *Preventive measure*
> Acquisition left-lateral planar image with patient in right side decubitus position.
> *Corrective measure*
> Repeat planar left lateral image with patient in right-side decubitus position.

## EQUILIBRIUM RADIONUCLIDE
## ANGIOCARDIOGRAPHY (FIG. 14-99 TO FIG. 14-106)

### ZOOM AND ACQUISITION OF VIEWS

ERNA images allow for interpretation of the morphology and contraction of the heart as well as the large vessels. In order to obtain optimal results, ERNA studies should be acquired with the appropriate zoom. The heart should not be too small or too large on the images. In addition to visualization of the right and left ventricle, a good quality ERNA also visualizes the aortic arch and pulmonary artery (9). Using a 13 in. diameter cardiac camera, the size of the heart should be about one-quarter to one-third of the diameter of the field of view.

Three planar projection images should be acquired for complete evaluation of the heart: supine anterior, supine left anterior oblique, and right-side decubitus left lateral (**Figs. 14-99** and **14-100**).

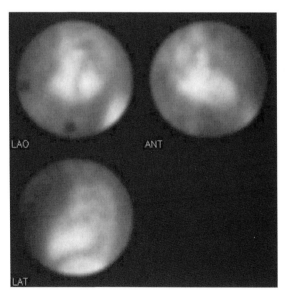

**Fig. 14-99.** Normal planar three-view ERNA study. The zoom factor should be such that the heart occupies about one-quarter to one-third of the field of view. All four chambers of the heart as well as the great vessels should be visible. This is a normal good quality study. The right atrium and right ventricle are normal in size and contraction. The left ventricle in slightly enlarged with normal regional wall motion. The great vessels are normal in shape.

## LABELING EFFICIENCY

Poor labeling of red blood cells may affect overall quality of ERNA images. However, free Tc-99m pertechnetate is usually trapped in thyroid gland, salivary glands, and stomach mucosa, and images may be of adequate interpretable quality. Poor quality of ERNA images is often due to body habitus. In overweight patients scattering of low-energy photons may significantly degrade image quality. Because the labeling of red cells is performed in vitro, there is a small chance of formation of small clumps of red blood cells. After injection of the radiolabeled red cells, the microclots may be trapped in the lungs and are visualized as multiple hot spots in the lungs (10). These clots are of microscopic size and of no clinical consequence.

## ECG-GATING PROBLEMS

The validity of information gained from ERNA studies depends on regular heart rate and appropriate ECG synchronization during acquisition. ECG-gating problems may be suspected by "blinking" during movie display of ERNA. The blinking is due to low total counts in the last frame(s) of ERNA. For purpose of display, technologists may remove frames with low counts from the end of the movie, resulting in display without blinking.

To assess the validity of image data and ejection fraction, one should inspect the generated left ventricular volume curve (6) Fig. 14-101. The "drop-off" in counts at the end of the curve indicates irregular heart rate during acquisition. As long as the ejection phase and end systole are not affected, calculated ejection fraction is accurate. An extreme example of heart rate irregularity is atrial fibrillation with a wide range of R-R intervals. In the latter condition an ERNA volume curve may have no well-defined end systole nadir. In the latter situation left ventricular ejection fraction cannot be calculated. In contrast, patients with atrial fibrillation and medically controlled heart rate may have a relatively narrow range of R-R intervals and (average) left ventricular ejection fraction can be calculated.

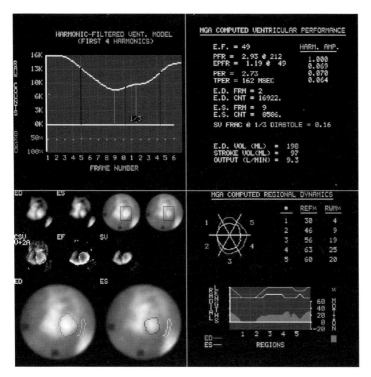

%**Fig. 14-100.** Computer screen display of processed data of the ERNA study shown in Fig. 14-99. The bottom panel at the left shows the end diastolic (ED) and end systolic (ES) regions of interest for calculation of ejection fraction (EF), as well as the crescent-shaped background region to the right of the left ventricular lateral wall. At the top in the same panel functional images are shown that may be used as guides for processing. The top panel on the left shows the count-based left ventricular volume curve. The curve has an appropriate physiologic shape. Diastolic filling appears to be relatively slow. The top right panel shows calculated parameters. EF is calculated to be low normal, 49%. Early peak filling rate (EPFR) is 1.19 ED volume/s. The counts in the ED frame (FRM) are 16,922 counts, ensuring good statistical reliability. The ED volume is enlarged at 198 mL. The bottom right panel shows values for regional ejection fraction (REF). Overall, this study shows normal right ventricular function. Slightly enlarged left ventricle with preserved low normal EF and decreased diastolic function.

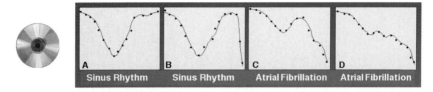

**Fig. 14-101.** Examples of count-based ERNA left ventricular volume curves in sinus rhythm and in atrial fibrillation. **(A)** Volume curve of a patient in sinus rhythm and perfect regular heart rate. After systole the volume curve returns to a similar end diastolic count level as at the beginning of the cardiac cycle. **(B)** Volume curve of a patient in sinus rhythm but irregular heart beats, either premature ventricular beats or marked respiratory variation. The last frames of the acquisition cycle were not always "filled" because of early R-waves prematurely stopping the acquisition. This is reflected as a drop-off in counts at the end of the volume curve. **(C)** Volume curve of a patient in atrial fibrillation and medically controlled heart rate. The drop-off in counts at the end of the volume curve is more marked due to variation in R-R intervals. A systolic trough is discernable and an "average" ejection fraction can be calculated. **(D)** Volume curve of a patient in atrial fibrillation without control of heart rate. There is a wide variation in R-R intervals. Numerous acquisition sequences are prematurely stopped. The volume curve slopes down and does not show a clear end systolic trough. Ejection fraction cannot be calculated.

## ERNA GATING PROBLEMS

*Recognition*
Blinking on movie display of ERNA.
Left ventricular volume curve with drop-off.
Left ventricular volume curve without clear systolic nadir.
*Preventive measure*
Acquire ERNA in patients with stable heart rate.
Acquire ERNA in list mode and reformat data.
Administer bolus of lidocaine IV unless contraindicated.
*Corrective measure*
Repeat ERNA acquisition when patient has regular heart rate.
Reformat list mode image data with selection of narrow RR interval.

## CALCULATION OF LEFT VENTRICULAR EJECTION FRACTION (LVEF) AND EFFECT OF BACKGROUND COUNTS

Left ventricular ejection fraction (LVEF) is derived from end diastolic (ED) counts, end systolic (ES) counts, and background counts (BKG) using the formula:

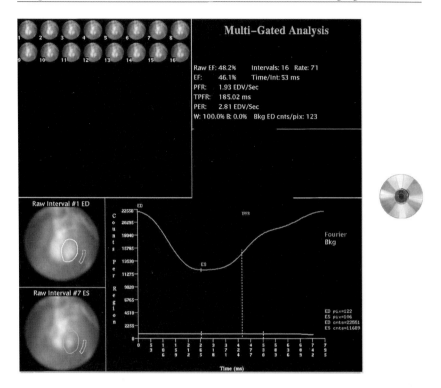

**Fig. 14-102.** This ERNA was processed using a fixed region of interest (ROI). The two images on the bottom left show the end diastolic (ED) image and the end systolic (ES) image. The ROI drawn over the left ventricle in ED is also used in the ES image. The ROI for background is shown in blue. Left ventricular ejection fraction (LVEF) is calculated as 46%. Using a fixed left ventricular ROI, noncardiac background activity is included in systolic counts and thus calculated LVEF is an underestimation of true LVEF.

$$\frac{(ED-BKG) - (ES-BKG)}{ED - BKG} = LVEF$$

For example, if BKG=0, ED=5000, ES=2000,

$$LVEF = \frac{5000-2000}{5000} = 0.60$$

LVEF determined using the above number is generally too low compared to a "gold standard" such as angiographic LVEF. To obtain an accurate value for LVEF, left ventricular counts must be corrected for background activity. The important effect of background subtraction is illustrated below: if BKG = 500,

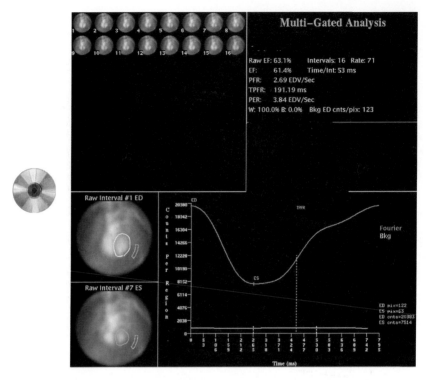

**Fig. 14-103.** Same ERNA as in Fig. 14-102. This time a variable ROI is used for calculation of LVEF. The ES ROI is smaller than the ED ROI and follows ES edges. The background ROI is placed in the same location as in Fig. 14-102. Thus, the only change is the ES ROI. Using a variable ROI LVEF is now 61%, which is the correct value for this patient.

$$\text{LVEF} = \frac{4500-1500}{4500} = 0.66$$

If BKG = 900,

$$\text{LVEF} = \frac{4100-1100}{4100} = 0.73$$

These example calculations show clearly that the higher background counts, the higher is the derived LVEF.

Because of the important effect of background selection on LVEF, the appropriate placement of the region of interest must always be checked before stating the value of LVEF in a final report.

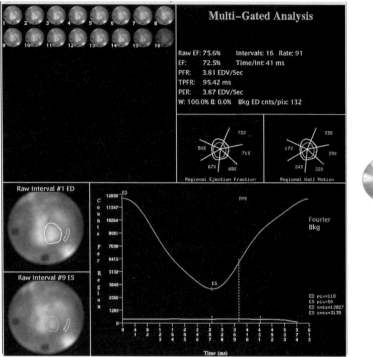

**Fig. 14-104.** Using correct processing parameters: variable ROIs over the left ventricle and background ROI to the right of the lateral in diastole, LVEF in this patient is 72%. Note the green line under the orange volume curve, which represents the level of background counts.

Background subtraction in processing ERNAs has been standardized by selecting the ROI as follows:

- Identify left ventricular end diastolic region of interest on LAO view.
- About 4 pixels off the lateral wall of the left ventricle in end diastole.
- A crescent-shaped region of interest about 4 pixel wide.
- About the height of the left ventricle.

**Figures 14-102** and **14-103** illustrate the effect of fixed and variable left ventricular regions of interest on calculated LVEF. **Figures 14-104, 14-105**, and **14-106** illustrate the effect of background selection on calculated LVEF.

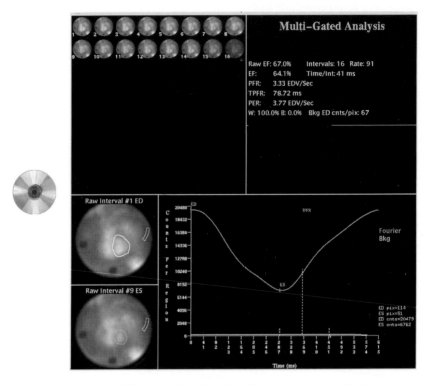

**Fig. 14-105.** Same ERNA as in Fig. 14-104. The same variable ROIs over the left ventricle are used as in Fig. 14-104. The background ROI is erroneously moved to the chest wall were background counts are lower. Note that the green background curve is lower than in Fig. 14-104. Using these ROIs LVEF is calculated to be 64%, which is too low.

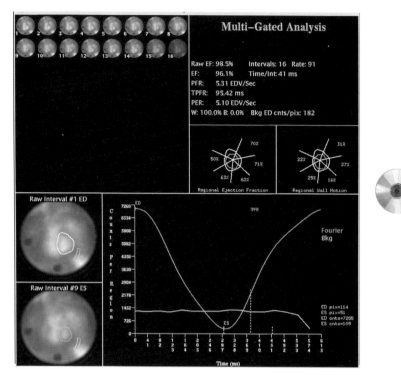

**Fig. 14-106.** Same ERNA as in Fig. 14-104. The same variable ROIs over the left ventricle are used as in Fig. 14-104. The background ROI is now erroneously moved to the spleen where background counts are higher. Note that the green background curve is substantially higher than in Fig. 14-104. Using these ROIs LVEF is calculated to be 96%, which is too high.

# SELECTED BIBLIOGRAPHY

1. Johnstone DE, Wackers FJTh, Berger HJ, et al. (1979). Effect of patient positioning on left lateral thallium-201 images. *J Nucl Med* 20:183–188.
2. Wackers F J Th (1992). Artifacts in planar and SPECT myocardial perfusion imaging. *Am J Cardiac Imaging* 6:42–58.
3. DePuey EG, Garcia EV (1989). Optimal specificity of thallium-201 SPECT through recognition of imaging artifacts. *J Nucl Med* 30:441.
4. DePuey EG, Rozanski A. (1995). Gated Tc-99m sestamibi SPECT to characterize fixed defects as infarct or artifact. *J Nucl Med* 36:952.
5. Hendel RC, Corbett JR, Cullom J, DePuey EG, Garcia EV (2002). The value and practice of attenuation correction for myocardial perfusion imaging: a joint position statement from the American Society of Nuclear Cardiology. *J Nucl Cardiol* 9:135–143.
6. King MA, Xia W, de Vries DJ, et al. (1996). A Monte Carlo investigation of artifacts caused by liver uptake in single photon emission computed tomography perfusion imaging with technetium-99m labele agents. *J Nucl Cardiol* 3:18.
7. Nichols K, Dorbala S, DePuey EG, Yao SS, Sharma A, Rozanski A (1999). Influence of arrhythmias on gated SPECT myocardial perfusion and function quantification. *J Nucl Med* 40:924–934.
8. Shen MYH, Liu Y, Sinusas AJ, et al. (1999). Quantification of regional myocardial wall thickening on ECG-Gated SPECT imaging. *J Nucl Cardiol* 6:583–595.
9. Wackers F J Th (1996). Equilibrium radionuclide angiocardiography. In Gerson MC (ed.), *Cardiac Nuclear Medicine*, 3rd Edition, Chapter 11. McGraw-Hill, New York, NY.
10. Benoit L, Wackers FJTh, Clements JP (1984). Clotting of Tc-99m labeled red cells. *J Nucl Med Tech* 12:59–60.

# 15 Nuclear Cardiology Reports

Until recently no standards for reporting results of nuclear cardiology studies existed. In 1997 the Intersocietal Commission for Accreditation of Nuclear Laboratories (ICANL) published standards and templates for optimal nuclear cardiology reports *(1)* (see www.icanl.org). The reason for this publication was that peer review of numerous laboratories revealed that the form, content, and quality of reports were highly variable and frequently poor. A poor quality report is at best of little value to the referring physician, and, at the worst, confusing, useless, and potentially harmful for patient care.

The most important purpose of a nuclear cardiology report is to communicate findings and clinical implications of stress tests and nuclear images to a referring physician. Thus, the report should help a referring physician in making clinical management decisions.

The referring physician is entitled to a clear conclusion: normal or abnormal, and if abnormal, how severely abnormal. The report may indicate, when appropriate, whether the risk for future cardiac events is low, moderate, or high. Certain imaging findings may have different clinical implications depending on the clinical context and results of stress testing. These nuances should be conveyed in an optimal report. If there were technical limitations to the study, they need to be stated and their impact on the final interpretation indicated. The second purpose of a report is to document for reimbursement purposes the services provided.

From: *Contemporary Cardiology: Nuclear Cardiology, The Basics*
F. J. Th. Wackers, W. Bruni, and B. L. Zaret © Humana Press Inc., Totowa, NJ

An adequate report should contain the following elements *(1–3)*:

- Patient demographics and ID number.
- Date of study.
- Summary of history.
- Indication for study.
- Type of stress and imaging test.
- (Radio)pharmaceutical(s) and dose(s).
- Stress findings, symptoms, ECG changes.
- Descriptive image interpretation.
- Final impression integrating stress and imaging findings.

Nuclear cardiology studies should be interpreted and reported on the day of performance. Final reports should be completed, signed, and mailed on average within 2 working days.

It is strongly recommended that abnormal test results be orally communicated to referring physicians on the day of performance of the test. This allows for a discussion of the results within the clinical context. Patients with markedly abnormal tests should not leave the imaging facility before the referring physician has been contacted.

The following templates for standardization (**Fig. 15-1–15-3**) of nuclear cardiology reports were published by the ICANL. These templates should be viewed as guidelines for form and content. Obviously reports can be individualized to one's personal style and needs.

In **Fig. 15-4** and **Fig. 15-5** examples of a *computer-generated report* and a *dictated report* on the same patient are shown. Both reports contain all elements required in an optimized report. **Figure 15-6** is a sample dictated report on an ERNA study of a different patient.

Fig. 15-1. (*right*) Template for standard exercise SPECT myocardial perfusion imaging report. Potential options to be communicated in the report are indicated within parentheses.

*Type of study:*
MYOCARDIAL PERFUSION IMAGING WITH *(SESTAMIBI/ TETROFOSMIN/ THALLIUM)*
SPECT AT REST AND AFTER EXERCISE, AND GATED SPECT *(,AND RESTING FIRST PASS RADIONUCLIDE ANGIOGRAPHY).*

*History:*
*(e.g. 65-yr woman with known coronary artery disease and recurrent chest pain).*

*Indication:*
*(e.g. Evaluation for coronary insufficiency; risk stratification; evaluation of ischemia; evaluation of functional capacity; evaluation of myocardial viability).*

*Procedure:*
The patient exercised on  treadmill (*bicycle*) for a total of ___ minutes, reaching stage ___ of the (*Bruce; modified Bruce, etc.*) protocol, achieving an estimated workload of ____ METs. The heart rate was ___ bpm at baseline, and increased to ___ bpm at peak exercise, representing 85% (*or ___ %*) of age-predicted maximal heart rate.  The blood pressure response was (*normal/ hypertensive/ hypotensive*). Resting blood pressure was ___mmHg, and peak/nadir blood pressure was ____mmHg.
The patient (*did/ did not*) have chest pain/symptoms during the procedure.
The electrocardiogram (*did not show/ showed*) ST-segment changes diagnostic for ischemia *(describe appropriate changes).*

The patient had myocardial perfusion imaging performed (*using a same day/ two day, dual isotope  imaging protocol)*, with the injection of ___mCi of (*radiopharmaceutical*) at peak exercise, and the injection of ___mCi of (*radiopharmaceutical e*) at rest.  Images were acquired by (*gated*) tomographic technique.

*Findings:*
The left ventricle was normal in size *(enlarged {degree of enlargement}/ LVH was present etc. Describe presence of transient dilation, if present. Describe increased post stress lung uptake, if present. Describe right ventricular abnormality, if present).*
There were no myocardial perfusion defects (*if abnormal describe: e.g.: there was a large antero-apical, antero-lateral perfusion defect on stress images, that was partially reversible on the rest images*).  *Mention whether artifacts were noted or suspected as well.*
By gated SPECT *(or by first pass angiography)* resting *(post exercise)* global resting LVEF was *normal/ abnormal.* LVEF was calculated (*or visually estimated*) at ___%.  Regional wall motion/thickening was normal, abnormal *(describe). (If appropriate one can describe right ventricular function from the gated SPECT study).*

*IMPRESSION:*
Normal *(or mildly abnormal, moderately abnormal, or markedly abnormal*) myocardial perfusion (*sestamibi/ tetrofosmin/ thallium-201*) SPECT imaging after (*excellent/ adequate/ fair/ submaximal*) exercise, showing a (*small/ moderate/ large*)  area of [*anatomic location*] infarction with or without (*small/ moderate/ large* ) amount of [*anatomic location*] ischemia.
*[If considered pertinent add the following info:]* The patients had (*yes or no*) symptoms. The stress ECG was *abnormal (describe).*  The hemodynamic response was *abnormal (describe).* Resting RV and LV function was (*normal/ abnormal*).

*[Add additional pertinent information that addresses the clinical reason for performing the study, such as low/high risk study. If appropriate mention suboptimal quality of study because of e.g. patient's obesity, etc].*

*Type of study:*
MYOCARDIAL PERFUSION IMAGING WITH (*SESTAMIBI/ TETROFOSMIN/ THALLIUM*)
SPECT AFTER VASODILATION WITH ADENOSINE *(DIPYRIDAMOLE, DOBUTAMINE)*, AND
GATED SPECT *(, AND RESTING FIRST PASS RADIONUCLIDE ANGIOGRAPHY)*.

*History:* As in figure 1. *Clarify why pharmacological stress was indicated, i.e. inability to exercise.*

*Indication:* As in figure 1.

*Procedure:*
The patient had a maximal dose of 140 mcg/kg/min of adenosine infused *(state if the patient also performed low level exercise). (If dipyridamole, give total dose infused over 4 minutes) (If dobutamine give maximal dose in mcg/kg/min).* The heart rate was ___bpm at baseline, and was ___bpm at peak adenosine/dipyridamole infusion. *(For dobutamine state maximal heart rate as percent of target heart rate).* The blood pressure response was (*normal/ hypertensive/ hypotensive*). [If blood pressure response was abnormal state: Resting blood pressure was ___mmHg, and peak/nadir blood pressure was ___mmHg].
The patient (*did/ did not*) have chest pain/symptoms during the procedure.
The electrocardiogram did *(did not) show* ST-segment changes suggestive of ischemia (describe changes if appropriate).

*Imaging procedure:* As in figure 1

*Findings:* As in figure 1

*IMPRESSION:* As in figure 1

**Fig. 15-2.** Template for standard vasodilator/adrenergic stress SPECT myocardial perfusion imaging report. Format as in Fig. 15-1.

*Type of study:*
EQUILIBRIUM RADIONUCLIDE ANGIOGRAPHY AT REST *(AND EXERCISE), (and gated first pass).*

*History:*
*(e.g. 74-yr male with lung cancer)*

*Indication: (e.g.assessment of global right ventricular/ left ventricular systolic/ diastolic function, regional wall motion, chemotherapy).*

*Procedure:*
The patient's red blood cells were labeled with ___mCi of Technetium-99m using the modified in vivo technique (using Ultratag etc). Imaging was performed at rest (and exercise) by planar technique in multiple views. *(By tomographic technique).*
*(If study is acquired during exercise describe type of exercise, duration, hemodynamic response, symptoms and ECG).*

*Findings:*
The right atrium was normal in size *(enlarged)*. The right ventricle was normal in size *(enlarged {degree of enlargement})*. Resting RVEF was ___%.
The pulmonary artery was normal in size *(dilated)*.
The left atrium was normal in size *(enlarged)*.
The left ventricle was normal in size *(enlarged {degree of enlargement})*. There was suggestion of left ventricular hypertrophy.
Regional wall motion was normal (*describe wall motion, paradoxical septal motion, hypokinesis {mild, moderate, severe}, akinesis, or dyskinetic segments*).
Global resting LVEF was normal (*mildly, moderately, severely reduced*) at ___%. *(During exercise LVEF was___ %)*
Resting end-diastolic volume was normal / *abnormal {i.e. mildly, moderately, severely enlarged)* at ___ mls.
Resting peak diastolic filling rate was normal *(abnormal)* at _____ end diastolic volumes/sec.


*IMPRESSION:*
Normal/ abnormal rest right ventricular function. Normal/abnormal resting left ventricular function. *(Normal/ abnormal LVEF response to exercise)*
*(Compare present assessment of LVEF to previous studies and comment)*

**Fig. 15-3.** Template for standard equilibrium radionuclide angiocardiography report. The format is as in Fig. 15-1.

**CARDIOVASCULAR NUCLEAR IMAGING AND EXERCISE LABORATORY**

Nuclear Cardiology          99 Main St.,  City, ST 99999          (999) 999-9999                    Rev. 4/02

## Patient

| | |
|---|---|
| Clinical history: | 60 year old white male with history of end stage ischemic cardiomyopathy.  Admitted with chest pain, shortness of breath post car accident.  CK/MB Troponin negative. |
| Indications: | Angina Pectoris (ICD-9: 413.9); Other forms of chronic ischemic heart disease (ICD-9: 414.8) |
| Asso.'d factors: | hypertension; smoking; hyperlipidemia; diabetes; known history of CAD;  ICD |
| Chest pain class: | atypical angina |
| Medications: | Metformin, Losartan, Torsemide, Gabapentin, Potassium Chloride,  Warfarin, Omeprazole, Allopurinol |
| Phys. Ex. -  Heart: | normal |
| - Lungs: | normal |
| | Weight: 280  lbs.      Height:  6  ft.   1  in. |
| Resting ECG: | sinus rhythm; Q waves- V1-5; Non-specific ST-T wave changes |

## Pharmacological Stress with Adenosine

Technique:   The patient underwent pharmacological stress with Adenosine at a maximum rate of 140 micrograms/kg/min.  (Total dose= 79.8 mg)

Rest HR:  70  bpm                Peak HR:  82  bpm

Rest BP: 100/78  mm Hg      Endpoint BP: 100/70  mm Hg      RPP/1000: 8.2  (adequate > 25)

Symptoms:  flushing

Termination:  protocol

ECG Changes:

**Fig. 15-4.** Sample of computer-generated report.

## CARDIOVASCULAR NUCLEAR IMAGING
## AND EXERCISE LABORATORY

| Nuclear Cardiology | 99 Main St., City, ST 99999 | (999) 999-9999 | Rev. 4/02 |

### Patient

### SPECT Myocardial Perfusion Imaging Following Adenosine Vasodilation and at Rest w Tc-99m Sestamibi with Gated SPECT and Analysis of Regional Wall Motion

The patient was injected with Tc-99m Sestamibi at peak stress (32.1 mCi) and at rest (30.2 mCi) and was studied with gated tomographic perfusion imaging.

*Findings:*

| | | |
|---|---|---|
| Lung Uptake: | normal |
| RV Size: | normal |
| LV Size: | enlarged LV |
| Artifact: | mild motion artifact |

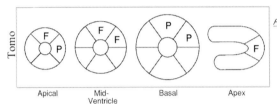

Tomo

Apical          Mid-          Basal          Apex
              Ventricle

*Perfusion defect code:*
"R"- reversible
"F"- fixed
"P"- partially reversible
"E"- equivocal
"X"- reverse redistribution
"D"- defect
"A"- artifact

### Perfusion Imaging Interpretation

*LV perfusion demonstrates:*   large mixed defect, predominantly scar

*Gated SPECT interpretation:*   LVEF:   44 %
Regional Wall Motion:   Anteroapical akinesis

### Stress Interpretation

Blood pressure response was normal. Chest pain was present. ECG changes were   nondiagnostic secondary to baseline ECG abnormality.

### Final Interpretation

Abnormal SPECT imaging after vasodilation with adenosine showing an enlarged LV with a large anterolateral and apical scar with a small amount of apical lateral ischemia. Global LVEF is depressed with anteroapical akinesis. Compared to previous studies there is no significant change.

*Read by:*
Frans J. Th. Wackers, M.D./ ejt

**DOE, JOHN**
**MRUN: 1234567**   DOB: Dec-02-1941    Report Date:  May-13-
2002
Cardiovascular Nuclear Imaging

Responsible Physician:
SMITH, JOHN  MD
CITY HOSPITAL
99 MAIN STREET
CITY, ST 99999


SPECT MYOCARDIAL PERFUSION IMAGING FOLLOWING ADENOSINE
VASODILATION AND AT REST WITH TC-99M SESTAMIBI WITH GATED
SPECT AND ANALYSIS OF REGIONAL WALL MOTION:  5/13/2002

CLINICAL HISTORY:
60 year old white male with history of end stage ischemic
cardiomyopathy.  Admitted with chest pain and shortness of
breath after a car accident.  Serial CK/MB and Troponin
were negative.

INDICATION:
Angina Pectoris; Chronic ischemic heart disease.

PROCEDURE:
The patient underwent pharmacological stress with
adenosine at a maximum infusion rate of 140
micrograms/kg/min (Total dose= 79.8 mg).  Resting heart
rate was 70 beats per minute and increased to 78 beats per
minute at peak adenosine infusion.  The blood pressure
response was normal: 100/78 mmHg at rest and 100/70 mmHg
at peak adenosine.  The patient developed chest pain
during adenosine infusion. There were non diagnostic
electrocardiographic changes during vasodilatory stress.
The patient had a two-day imaging protocol and was
injected with 32.1 mCi of Sestamibi at peak adenosine
infusion and 30.2 mCi of Sestamibi at rest. Imaging was
performed by ECG-gated tomographic technique.

FINDINGS:
The lung uptake for this study was normal.  The right
ventricle was normal in size.  The left ventricle was
enlarged.  Myocardial perfusion imaging demonstrated a
large fixed anterolateral and apical defect with small
reversiblity in the same area, in particular at the base.
Interpretation of this study was complicated by mild
motion artifact. By gated SPECT, global left ventricular
ejection fraction was moderately depressed at 44% with
anteroapical akinesis.

**Fig. 15-5.** Sample of dictated report on the same patient as in Fig. 15-4.

```
SMITH, JANE
MRUN: 0123456   DOB: JUL-22-1945   Report Date: NOV-19-2002

DIAGNOSTIC IMAGING CONSULTATION

        Responsible Physician:
            SMITH, JOHN   MD
            CITY HOSPITAL
            CITY, ST 9999
---------------------------------------------------------------
--


EQUILIBRIUM RADIONUCLIDE ANGIOGRAPHY:   11/19/2002

CLINICAL HISTORY:
57 year old female presents with syncope, here for
cardiac
evaluation.

INDICATION:
Acute ischemic heart disease

PROCEDURE:
The patient's red blood cells were labeled with 32.1 mCi
of technetium using the Ultratag technique.  Imaging was
performed by the planar technique in multiple views.

FINDINGS:
The right atrium was normal in size.  The right ventricle
was normal in size.  Right ventricular function was
normal.  The left atrium was normal in size.  The left
ventricle was enlarged.  The left ventricular ejection
fraction was markedly depressed at 33%. End diastolic
volume was abnormal at 250 cc.  There was also dilation
of the aorta.  Regional wall motion was abnormal with
anteroapical-septal hypokinesis.

IMPRESSION:
Normal right ventricular function. Abnormal left
ventricular function with an enlarged left ventricle,
depressed LVEF, and anteroapical and septal regional wall
motion abnormality. This study is consistent with
ischemic cardiomyopathy.

I have reviewed the images and dictated/reviewed/or
edited the final
(signed)      Frans Wackers, MD
```

**Fig. 15-6.** Sample of dictated report on an ERNA study of a different patient.

# SELECTED BIBLIOGRAPHY

1. Wackers F J Th (2000). Intersocietal Commission for the Accreditation of Nuclear Medicine Laboratories (ICANL) Position Statement on Standardization and Optimization of Nuclear Cardiology Reports. *J Nucl Cardiol* 7:397–400.
2. Cerqueira MD (1996). The user-friendly nuclear cardiology report: what needs to be considered and what needs to be included. *J Nucl Cardiol* 3:350–355.
3. Hendel RC, Wackers FJ Th, Berman DS, Ficaro E, DePuey EG, Tilkemeyer P, Klein L, Cerqueira M (2004). Reporting of radionuclide myocardial perfusion imaging studies, ASNC Position Statement. *J Nucl Cardiol* (in press).

# 16 Remote Reading and Networking

## *Tele-Nuclear Cardiology*

Remote interpretation of nuclear cardiology images by electronic means or *tele-nuclear cardiology* may be very useful for two reasons. It is not unusual at the present time for a nuclear cardiology laboratory to provide interpretation for one or more remote satellite imaging facilities *(1)*. These facilities operate generally under the same technical and medical directors, but are geographically distant and may have their own local technical staff. Second, even if there is only one laboratory, for reasons of competitiveness, an imaging facility may be required to provide service outside routine office hours. Under these conditions, it is very desirable to create a technical environment that allows for remote interpretation through tele-nuclear cardiology. Recently, guidelines have been published that address procedures, quality assurance, and security for tele-nuclear medicine *(2)* (on line: www.snm.org/policy/new_guidelines_1.html).

---

Tele-nuclear cardiology can be achieved in a number of ways as described in brief in this chapter.

## MODES OF COMMUNICATION

One has to consider various modes of electronic communication and transfer of image data. Several media can be used to connect two remote locations; from slower to faster connectivity speed, they are

- By modem and regular phone line (56kbps).
- ISDN (integrated services digital network) line (112kbps).
- DSL (digital subscriber line) (1.5Mbps).

From: *Contemporary Cardiology: Nuclear Cardiology, The Basics*
F. J. Th. Wackers, W. Bruni, and B. L. Zaret © Humana Press Inc., Totowa, NJ

- Digital cable modem (1Gbps).
- T1 line (1 Gbps).

One should also consider whether one intends to use a personal computer as a remote workstation or merely as a viewing terminal. The electronic connection can be established:

1. Between a computer in the main nuclear cardiology laboratory and a remote computer in a satellite laboratory, or
2. Between a computer in the main nuclear cardiology laboratory and a remote personal computer at the physician's home, or a remote laptop computer while the physician is travelling.

Three practical options should be considered.

- First option: The remote computer dials in through one of the above-mentioned connectivity media with the digital environment in the main nuclear cardiology laboratory. Using Window emulator software (e.g., X-Window Emulator or PC-Anywhere®), the physician can review processed image data. In this configuration the home computer serves as a viewing terminal for the main computer in the laboratory.
- Second option: Once a connection with the main laboratory has been established, raw image data are downloaded through one of the above connectivity means to the remote workstation, which has all the processing and display software required for offline data processing, image viewing, and interpretation. In this configuration the home computer becomes another workstation of the laboratory.

These two options are both somewhat cumbersome and in our view not optimal. The speed of access and of viewing using the first option may be relatively slow, but the physician does not have to (re)process any image data. The speed of the second option depends largely on the quantity of data to be downloaded. For example, the downloading of complete data of an ECG-gated SPECT study may be very time-consuming. Furthermore, the physician has to perform all data processing by him/herself.

- Third option: Web reading

  We consider this the most practical solution. The physician interprets nuclear cardiology images on a secure internet website. Reconstructed and processed images are uploaded by a technologist from the nuclear medicine computer in the main laboratory to a dedicated website as simple compressed image files, e.g., gif, tiff, jpeg, png, bmp, or mpeg cine files. One can also upload scanned files of technologists' worksheets, rest/stress ECGs, and other relevant written data as PDF files. The website is accessed by the physician from the remote computer through the internet and a commercial web browser. The physician can then either view the images on the website or download data to the personal computer. The advantage of "web reading" is its simplicity and speed of access. In our experience even a regular phone line provides acceptable speed. A minor disadvantage of this method is that the interpreter cannot (re)process images if he/she desires to do so. However, standardization of processing and display should make this unnecessary most of the time.

## QUALITY ASSURANCE

As with every other procedure in radionuclide imaging, a number of QA issues should be considered for tele-nuclear cardiology.

### *The Integrity and Preservation of Images*

It is conceivable, although rare, that during transfer of raw or processed images, corruption of data occurs. Also, too much compression of images for uploading to the website may deteriorate image quality. These potential problems should be evaluated by empirical testing of a number of different compressed file formats. Original image data should be compared qualitatively and quantitatively to the digitally transferred data on the receiving computer.

### *Speed*

The speed of access and the speed of viewing individual images are extremely important in clinical practice. For example, if it takes longer than 45–60 s to download or display one single image, the entire process of remote reading becomes extremely tedious. In particular, if multiple patient studies are to be interpreted, reasonable speed is crucial.

### *Security*

Patients confidentiality and security have become extremely important with the new HIPAA regulations. Incoming and outgoing patient data must be encrypted and should be accessible only by authorized users with username and password, and must be in compliance with HIPAA regulations.

What is HIPAA?

The Health Insurance Portability & Accountability Act (HIPAA) of 1996 (August 21), Public Law 104-191, which amends the Internal Revenue Service Code of 1986. Also known as the Kennedy–Kassebaum Act.

Title II includes a section, "Administrative Simplification", requiring:

1. Improved efficiency in healthcare delivery by standardizing electronic data interchange, and
2. Protection of confidentiality and security of health data through setting and enforcing standards.

More specifically, HIPAA calls for:

1. Standardization of electronic patient health, administrative, and financial data
2. Unique health identifiers for individuals, employers, health plans, and health care providers
3. Security standards protecting the confidentiality and integrity of "individually identifiable health information," past, present, or future.

For more information see: http://www.hipaadvisory.com

Telemedicine can be viewed as communication of Protected Health Information (PHI) between "Business Associates." The HIPAA Business Associate standard mandates that Business Associates who may receive, use, obtain, create, or have access to PHI be required to sign an agreement that will ensure that the Business Associate will safeguard and protect the integrity and confidentiality of the PHI.

## *Quality of Remote Display*

In order to have diagnostic quality images, the remote display monitor should have similar resolution and quality of display as those of the computers in the main nuclear cardiology imaging facility (e.g., 1024 × 768 resolution and true color).

## LOCAL COMPUTER NETWORK

When there are multiple gamma cameras in a nuclear cardiology imaging facility, a local area network (LAN) is useful for making daily operation easier and more efficient. The images acquired on different acquisition computers are transferred through the LAN to a central computer for either central processing and/or for central display in a reading room.

The typical hardware components of a LAN are

- Main computer with network software and Ethernet card.
- Hub.
- Router.
- RJ45 cables for inter-computer connections.
- Fire wall for protection from intrusion from outside.

## STORAGE

Storage of digital image data (raw and/or processed data) is of clinical importance because it allows for comparison of a recent patient study with previous studies of the same patient. Raw image data may be transferred from the acquisition computers through the LAN to a central computer that serves as a storage device. For easy access to previous studies, it is advisable to store relatively recent (< 3 yr) data on-line for a limited number of years. For long-term storage, image data can be stored on optical disks and/or tapes. Obviously retrieval of data from optical disks , and, in particular, from magnetic tape, takes considerably more time than on-line retrieval. In our laboratory all data are doubly backed up in storage. For storage of large volumes of digital data, storage on juke-box and raid library is an optimal solution. For accreditation by the ICANL, it is a requirement that one submits digital data retrieved from storage.

## SELECTED BIBLIOGRAPHY

1. Bateman TM, Cullom J, Case JA (1999). Wide area networking in nuclear cardiology. *J Nucl Cardiol* 6:211–218.
2. Parker JA, Wallis JW, Jadvar H, Christian P, Todd-Pokropek A (2002). Procedure guideline for telenuclear medicine 1.0. *J Nucl Med* 43:1410–1413.

# 17 Quality Assurance

Ongoing quality assurance is a vital component for the optimal functioning of a laboratory. All equipment, including imaging and nonimaging equipment, must be checked regularly to ensure proper functioning. In addition to the technical quality assurance of equipment, it is recommended that a program is in place that periodically assesses the quality of technologists and interpreting staff.

The following are some common definitions used in quality assurance:

- Quality Control (QC): Assessment of the proper performance of instrumentation
- Quality Assurance(QA): Assessment of all variables that are involved in the overall functioning of the laboratory
- Continuing Quality Improvement (CQI): Process of repeatedly setting new targets for improved performance of one of the aspects of QA

Standard QC protocols are described in detail in the Updated Imaging Guidelines for Nuclear Cardiology Procedures (*J Nucl Cardiol* 8:G1–G58, 2001, or on line: www.asnc.org; menu: library and resources: guidelines and standards).

## CAMERA QUALITY CONTROL

One must refer to the manufacturer's instructions for specific acquisition details and recommended frequencies of QC. Table 17-1 lists some important items for camera QC. The following subsections discuss the individual items.

### *Uniformity (Figs. 17-1 to 17-3)*

A high-count uniformity flood (30 million counts) is acquired either monthly or quarterly, depending on the manufacturer's recommenda-

From: *Contemporary Cardiology: Nuclear Cardiology, The Basics*
F. J. Th. Wackers, W. Bruni, and B. L. Zaret © Humana Press Inc., Totowa, NJ

## Table 17-1
## Variables to be Checked for Camera Quality Control (QC)

| QC | Frequency |
| --- | --- |
| Uniformity | Daily (2–6 million counts) |
| Energy peaking | Daily |
| Linearity | Weekly |
| Center of rotation | Monthly |
| High count uniformity | Monthly (30 million counts) |
| Preventive maintenance | 6 mo |

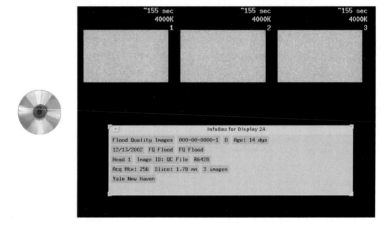

**Fig. 17-1.** Example of daily floods (approx 4,000,000 counts) of a triple-head gamma camera. All three heads are well-tuned and show good uniformity.

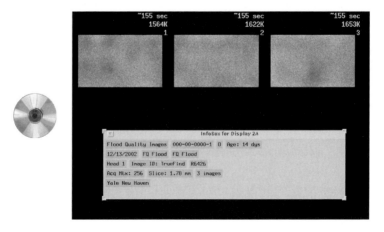

**Fig. 17-2.** Example of uncorrected daily floods (approx 1,500,000 counts) of a triple-head gamma camera. Non-uniformity is noted for each head. This was less than 5% and should be corrected for clinical use.

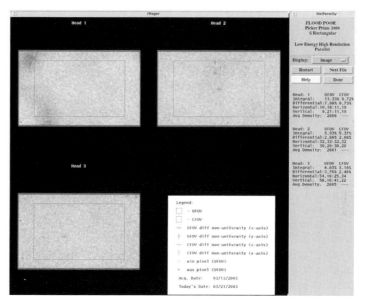

**Fig. 17-3.** Daily floods of a triple-head camera. The center field of view (CFOV) is marked by the red-lined rectangle in the center of the useable field of view (UFOV). The small circles and squares indicate pixels used for uniformity calculations. Head 1 has marked nonuniformity. Head 2 has minor nonuniformity. Head 3 shows good uniformity. For Head 1 integral uniformity of the UFOV is 13.3% and that of the CFOV is 9.7%. Both should be less than 5%. The vendor of this camera recommends that the calculation of the integral uniformity is used rather than of differential uniformity. For Head 2 UFOV and CFOV uniformity is marginal at 5.53% and 5.37%. The area of nonuniformity can clearly be appreciated in the upper middle-half of the UFOV. Gamma camera service should be called to correct the problem before a patient can be imaged with this camera.

tions. A high-count uniformity flood should be done for each type of collimator used and for each isotope commonly used in the laboratory. However, it should be noted that on some older systems (over 10 yr old), only one high-count uniformity flood is capable of being stored. In these cases, by necessity, only one uniformity flood is applied to the different isotopes acquired. While this is not ideal, storing one uniformity flood is an inherent limitation of the older imaging systems. Cameras under 10 yr of age usually require a separate high-count uniformity flood for each isotope. Check with the manufacturer for details.

High-count uniformity floods can be done extrinsically or intrinsically similar to the daily floods. It is usually recommended acquiring extrinsic floods in order to correct for irregularities of the collimator.

Because the required number of counts for these high-count floods is very high (30 million counts), they are often acquired overnight and analyzed in the morning. For a multiple-headed camera system, it may take a number of hours to acquire the uniformity flood.

---

QC of daily uniformity flood (2–6 million counts) can be done *extrinsically* or *intrinsically*.

An *extrinsic flood* is usually done with a Co-57 sheet source, or fillable flood source with Tc-99m, Tl-201, or any other isotope used in the laboratory. The source is placed on the detector's collimator. A static image is acquired and then analyzed for uniformity. Each vendor may have different acquisition parameters, and one should check with the manufacturer for specific recommendations. Most systems have an automatic program for analyzing the static image for percent uniformity. Again, each manufacturer will have different uniformity tolerance limits. It is recommended that one always visually inspect the image for hot and cold areas, indicating nonuniformity. A daily log should kept to record the percent uniformity daily. This allows one to look for slow drifts in uniformity.

*Intrinsic floods* are done with a Tc-99m point source with a small volume (0.5 mL) and low activity (100–200 μCi) acquired with the collimator off the gamma camera detector head. A static image is acquired and then analyzed for uniformity. Just as with extrinsic floods it is recommended that one visually inspect the image for hot and cold areas indicating nonuniform areas. Daily percent uniformity should be recorded in a log. If any problems with the uniformity are noted, camera service should be called in immediately.

---

Two parameters are used to measure and document flood uniformity:

*Integral uniformity*: This is a global parameter that measures contrast over an extended area of the detector and is expressed as percentage [$100\% \times (max-min)/(max+min)$].

*Differential uniformity*: This is a regional parameter that measures contrast over a small area. The measurement is performd using a $5 \times 1$ pixel area in both the X and Y directions and is expressed as percentage ($100\% \times$ largest deviation $(max-min)/(max+min)$).

*Both percentages must be* < 5%. (Max = maximal count found in any pixel within the specified area; min = mimimal count found in any pixel within the specified area.)

## *Energy Peaking*

On many newer model cameras, energy peaking is done automatically with the daily flood. Even if the computer program performs the analysis, one must check that the peak is within specified limits. A pulse height analysis (PHA) or digital readout should be checked daily to make sure that the peak is centered. The peak should be recorded daily to watch for drifts in the peak.

If peaking is not an automated part of the daily flood set-up, one should check the peak manually. All systems provide a visual display of the PHA and will allow adjusting the peak as necessary. Service should be notified of any drifts in the peak.

Incorrect peaking, either too high or too low, may affect field uniformity as shown in **Fig. 17-4**.

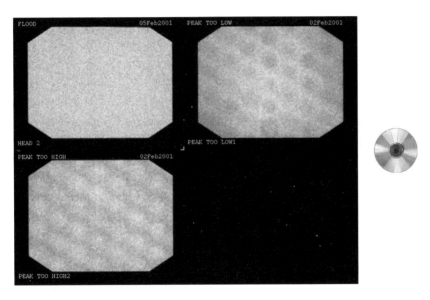

**Fig. 17-4.** Example of the effect of energy peaking on field flood uniformity. By peaking either too low (upper right) or too high (lower left) relative to the energy peak marked non-uniformity results which may affect clinical imaging.

## *Linearity (Figs. 17-5, 17-6)*

Linearity is more commonly known as "acquiring a bar flood." A bar phantom (phantom with variously sized lead bars) is placed on the collimator and the Co-57 sheet source is placed on top of the phantom. A

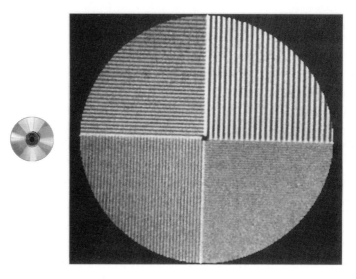

**Fig. 17-5.** Bar phantom. All lines are straight, indicating appropriate linearity. The bar phantom can also be used as a quick check on resolution. In the phantom shown, the lines in three of four quadrants are well separated and visible. Even smallest bars can be made out as a linear pattern, although they are not clearly separated. For daily QC it is important to document *and record* gradual changes in camera performance.

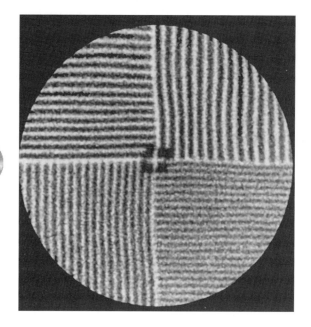

**Fig. 17-6.** Bar phantom showing wavy poor linearity. Nevertheless, resolution is apparently not affected. The gamma camera needs to be tuned-up by the vendor's maintenance service.

static image is acquired and visually inspected to make sure all of the bars are visible and that they are straight. Any "waviness" of the lines should be reported to service immediately.

## CENTER OF ROTATION (FIGS. 17-7, 17-8)

This measures the alignment error between the electronic matrix of the detector and the mechanical center of rotation. Depending on manufacturer recommendations, the center of rotation (COR) should be tested monthly or quarterly. To assess COR offset, SPECT acquisition of a Tc-99m point source is performed. The half-width-full-maximum of the reconstructed image of the point source is measured and analyzed to make sure that the COR has not drifted. Each manufacturer will have different acquisition parameters and different acceptable values. If the COR is not within the recommended range, the gamma camera should not be used and service must be called immediately. COR errors can cause serious image artifacts. In general COR offset should not exceed 2 pixels using a $64 \times 64$ matrix. COR offset affects image resolution and causes image blurring.

### *Preventive Maintenance*

It is usually recommended that service be scheduled every 6 mo for preventive maintenance of the camera and computer system. Depending on the gamma camera and whether any defaults have to be corrected, this usually takes 4–8 h to complete. Having imaging equipment inoperable for any length of time is a burden on the daily operation of the imaging facility; but *scheduled* maintenance is easier to tolerate than an unexpected breakdown of a gamma camera. Not infrequently, preventive maintenance detects technical problems before they become a clinical problem.

## NON-IMAGING EQUIPMENT QC

Table 17-2 lists some important items for non-imaging equipment QC. The following subsections discuss the individual items.

### *Dose Calibrator Constancy*

The dose calibrator must be checked each working day prior to use. A Cs-137 source is normally used for this purpose. The standard known source is measured daily in the dose calibrator. The daily measurements should be recorded. The radiation safety officer usually provides a table with ranges of measured activities for any given day. Since the Cs-137 source decays, the range will change continually. The measurements of

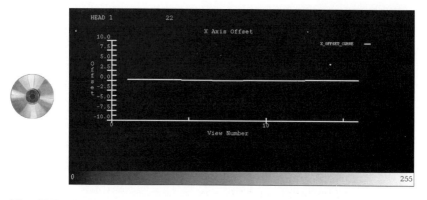

**Fig. 17-7.** Display of center-of rotation (COR) offset testing results. The offset is plotted against acquisition angles. The COR is within acceptable range.

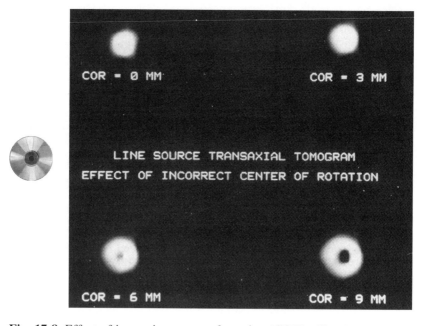

**Fig. 17-8.** Effect of increasing center of rotation (COR) offset (expressed in mm) on reconstructed image of a line source. The image is increasingly blurred by circular smearing with increasing COR offset. Ultimately, at 9 mm offset (about 4 pixels) the line source is reconstructed as a circle. COR offset results in loss of image resolution.

Cs-137 activity must fall within the daily predefined range and thus confirm that the dose calibrator functions properly.

### Table 17-2
### Non-imaging Equipment QC

| QC | Frequency |
| --- | --- |
| **Dose calibrator** | |
| Constancy | Daily |
| Accuracy | Quarterly |
| Linearity | Quarterly |
| **Survey meter** | |
| Source check | Daily |
| Calibration | Yearly |
| **Treadmills and ECG equipment** | |
| Electrical safety | Yearly |

## *Dose Calibrator Accuracy*

In addition to the daily QC check, the dose calibrator should undergo quarterly QC requirements. To perform the accuracy test of the dose calibrator, one needs four known standard sources Co-57, Co-60, Cs-137, and Ba-133 are commonly used for this test. Each source is measured in the dose calibrator and the activity is recorded. The radiation safety officer should set acceptable measured ranges of activities for each radioisotope.

## *Dose Calibrator Linearity*

The second quarterly required QC test of the dose calibrator is a linearity test. One draws a known amount of Tc-99m (usually around 100 mCi) in a vial and periodically measures and records the measured activity of the vial as it decays. Typically two to three measurements per day are taken until the source has decayed to 30 μCi. The radiation safety officer can again be of assistance in determining whether the measurements are within acceptable limits.

## QUALITY ASSURANCE AND CONTINUING QUALITY IMPROVEMENT

Quality assurance is a program for the systematic monitoring and evaluation of various aspects of a project, service, or facility to ensure that standards of quality are being met. It is an important process that allows for timely identification of problems or areas of improvement, facilitates the initiation of necessary changes in policies or procedures, and improves efficiency. Table 17-3 lists some QA terminology.

**Table 17-3**
**QA Terminology**

| | |
|---|---|
| Indicator | Predefined item that is being assessed |
| Threshold | Limit tolerated before action is needed and beyond which the situation is unacceptable |
| Corrective action | Measure used to correct the problem and return to within the threshold |

## In order to begin a QA program:

- Support of the medical director or manager is required
- Decide what area needs QA, i.e.
    Problem area
    Uncertain status in an area
- Define what information or data are needed
- Determine limits or thresholds
- Determine corrective action to be taken to fix the problem
- Write a protocol including thresholds and corrective actions
- Create form or worksheet for the collection of data
- Make data collection part of laboratory routine (for future re-evaluations)
- Take the corrective action and fix the problem

---

**Possible suggested areas for QA include the following:**

- Technical issues
    - Reproducibility
    - Poor quality studies
    - Service call response times
    - Camera downtime
    - Camera quality control
- Safety
    - Misadministrations
    - Radioisotope spills
    - Inadvertent needle sticks (staff)
    - Patient incidents
    - Staff incidents
- Efficiency
    - Patient wait times
    - Exam backlog
    - Camera usage
- Satisfaction
    - Patient satisfaction
    - Referring physician satisfaction
- Interpretation
    - Reviewer reproducibility
    - Comparison to another modality
- Reporting
    - Timeliness of report generation
    - Timeliness of signing
    - Timeliness of mailing
    - Transcription errors
    - Quantity of errors

---

The above table lists only some suggested areas. There are numerous other aspects of the operation of a laboratory that can be submitted to QA. It is important to remember that a QA program should be an individualized process. Those aspects addressed by a QA program in one laboratory may not necessarily be relevant for another laboratory. Ultimately a QA program should result in an improvement of services. Every individual laboratory may have specific needs. For instance, detailed documentation of downtime of an old camera may be used as a persuasive argument for replacing old equipment.

# 18 Miscellaneous Additional Laboratory Protocols and Policies

Every nuclear cardiology imaging facility should have written protocols for all procedures. In addition, written protocols and policies should be in place for all other medical and nonmedical procedures and anticipated incidents.

Protocols and policies should be easily available to the staff, i.e., a copy should be present in the imaging rooms or stress laboratory. Many hospital protocols and policies are posted on the hospital's web site. These policies not only help to run a laboratory more efficiently, but also prepare them for dealing with potential problems. Safety should be a major concern for any laboratory. The policies listed in this chapter are also required by the ICANL for accreditation of a nuclear cardiology laboratory ( see also www.icanl.org).

A nuclear cardiology imaging facility should have at the minimum written protocols and policies for the following:

- Radiation safety and handling of radiopharmaceuticals
- Clinical indications of procedures
- Medical emergencies
- Patient identification
- Patient pregnancy assessment
- Patient confidentiality and HIPAA compliance
- Infection control
- Electrical equipment safety
- Fire safety

Protocols should be dated and preferably signed by the medical and technical director.

From: *Contemporary Cardiology: Nuclear Cardiology, The Basics*
F. J. Th. Wackers, W. Bruni, and B. L. Zaret © Humana Press Inc., Totowa, NJ

## Radiation Safety and Handling of Radiopharmaceuticals

These written protocols are extremely important. Radiation safety must be taken seriously. Every imaging facility should have a radiation safety officer and written policies on the receipt and storage of radioisotopes/radiopharmaceuticals, proper preparation and calibration of radiopharmaceuticals, proper administration of radiopharmaceuticals, disposal of the radioactive trash, and how to handle spills of radiotracer. The policies should also discuss the proper use and quality control of radiation safety equipment and techniques to reduce technologist radiation exposure.

## Clinical Indications

The clinical indications for stress testing and imaging procedures should be in compliance with the published AHA/ACC guidelines.

## Cardiac Emergency

A written protocol should be in place for cardiac emergencies. In general, exercise testing is very safe. Using the Bruce, modified Bruce, or other standardized graded protocols, cardiac emergencies (persistent severe ischemia, acute infarction, cardiac death) occur infrequently (1:10,000 exercise tests). However, with an increasingly sicker patient population and greater number of patients with known coronary artery disease referred for study, cardiac emergencies may occur more frequently. Consequently, laboratory personnel should be well prepared to deal with cardiac emergencies.

A qualified health care provider, certified in CPR or ACLS, should supervise and be responsible for stress testing. As a rule two people are needed to administer an exercise test. Defibrillation equipment and "crash cart" must be present in the immediate vicinity of the stress laboratory. Laboratory personnel (including technologists and administrative personnel) should know what to do when a "code" is called.

In order to deal adequately with emergencies all exercise staff and preferably also imaging staff should know:

1. Emergency phone number(s).
2. Where emergency equipment and medications, i.e., crash cart, are located.
3. How to assemble the Ambu bag and hook up to oxygen.
4. How to turn on the defibrillator and place chest leads.
5. How to start CPR.
6. How to assist physician(s) and nurse(s) during CPR.

## Patient Identification

Every laboratory should have a policy on how to properly identify or confirm a patient's identity. In a hospital laboratory in-patients usually wear ID bracelets that should be used to verify identity. For out-patients it is not sufficient to just call a patient's name in the waiting area. There have been many instances where a patient misunderstood the name called and answered to the wrong name. The written protocol should specify that a patient's identity should also be checked by verifying date of birth or social security number.

## Patient Pregnancy Assessment

All women of childbearing years should be asked whether or not they might be pregnant or breastfeeding prior to beginning the stress or imaging procedure. The protocol should include under what age a women should be asked if she is pregnant or breastfeeding, what to do if she answers "may be, or I don't know," and what to do if she indicates that she is pregnant or breastfeeding .

## Patient Confidentiality

All patient records and information must be kept confidential and each laboratory should have a written policy in place on how this issue is ensured. Patient confidentiality has become extremely important with the new HIPAA regulations (see Chapter 16).

## Electrical Equipment Safety

All electrical equipment should be checked annually to ensure that it is safe to use. A written policy on what to do if unsafe electrical equipment is found and how to use electrical equipment properly is recommended.

## Fire Safety

A written policy on what to do in the case of a fire is highly recommended. The policy should include how to use a fire extinguisher, who to contact in case fire or smoke is detected, what steps to take to contain the fire, and what is the best evacuation route.

## Infection Control

Control of infection is an important concern in hospitals and in out-patient facilities . A written policy on how to use properly universal precautions should be in place. The policy should discuss the use of gloves, aseptic techniques, and proper disposal of biohazardous trash.

# EXAMPLES

The following are illustrative examples of written policies from our laboratory (see also the ICANL website www.icanl.org)

## *Example 1. Dose Calibration and Administration*

- Every radioactive kit prepared must have a Dose Log Sheet.
- The log sheet must contain the radiopharmaceutical, date, total activity in kit in mCi, total volume used in kit, concentration (activity in mCi/volume in mL), and time the kit was prepared.
- Every patient dose must be logged on the Dose Log Sheet with patient name, procedure (Stress or Rest), and time.
- To calculate the concentration at the time of injection:
  Take the original concentration and multiply by the decay factor (Tc-99m decay chart hanging on bulletin board).
- To calculate how much isotope to draw up:
  Dose desired (mCi) / new concentration (mCi/mL) = volume to draw up (mL).
- Assay the dose in the dose calibrator.
- Adjust the dose as necessary to get the desired dose.
- Label the dose with the patient name, activity, time, and isotope.
- Record actual dose drawn up on Dose Log Sheet.
- Important: A patient can only be injected with ± 10% of the desired dose. If the dose is adjusted for the patients weight, note on the log sheet and refer to the Tc-99m Adjusted Dose Chart.
- Pediatric patients (< 18 yr old) must have their dose adjusted for their weight using the following formula:

[weight (lb) / 150 (lb)] × adult dose

example: child of 50 lb, usual adult dose = 25 mCi

thus, (50 lb /150 lb) × 25 mCi = 8.33 mCi to be given to this child

Note: nonstandard dosing should be given only after consultation with the nuclear cardiologist.

- All doses should be carried in a lead carrying case or lead pig. All doses should be in a lead syringe shield during injection.
- All injections are done through a three-way tubing for rest and exercise tests, or a Y-connector for adenosine and dobutamine tests.
- The port should be swabbed with an alcohol pad prior to injection.
- Rest and exercise injections should be flushed with 10 cc of normal saline.

- Adenosine and dobutamine injections should be flushed with 4 cc of normal saline.
- All needles, syringes, and gloves must be placed in appropriate hot trash receptacles.

Revised October 2002

## Example 2. Hot Trash Policy

- Hot trash is to be collected, boxed, stored, and discarded every week. All needle boxes should have tops on and all red bags should be tied closed. Wear gloves when dealing with any potential radioactive material or trash. Please review the following checklist when storing and/or discarding hot trash.
- Place all needle boxes and red bags in black biohazard boxes
- Survey the decay room and hallway and record the measurements in the appropriate section of the decay log book (located in the inner decay room on the shelf)
- Label the boxes with the date and the next available log number (ex. C###). Boxes containing needle boxes must be labeled SHARPS.
- Record the date and the log number of each box in the decay log book.
- Record the potential discard date of the boxes (TWO months from the storage date!!)
- See if any previously stored boxes can be discarded.
- Survey the boxes to be discarded and record the measurements and the date in the decay log book. (If they are not equal to background or less, they CAN NOT be discarded!)
- Take the boxes to be discarded (..location..) and label as "trash."

Revised October 2002

## Example 3. Patient Pregnancy Assessment

- Nuclear technologists will ask all female patients under 50 years of age if they are or might be pregnant or are breast feeding.
- If the patient answers No, it MUST be recorded in the computerized hospital information system or worksheet for documentation. For example: Patient states not pregnant/breast feeding. Initial and date the statement.
- A pregnancy test will be administered if a patient states they do not know or might be pregnant. Negative results will be recorded on the

CCSS or worksheet for documentation. For example: Patient given urine pregnancy test and a negative result was obtained. Initial and date the statement.

Urine pregnancy test

- Have the patient urinate into a paper cup
- Open a pregnancy test kit and fill the dropper with urine
- Fill the corner hole on the kit from the dropper with urine until the paper is saturated
- Wait approx 60 s, or until the display hole turns completely pink.
  If a – sign appears, the patient is NOT pregnant
  If a + sign appears, the patient IS pregnant
- The technologist will inform the physician if a patient is pregnant.
- The physician will contact the referring physician to consult in the decision to proceed with the exam, limit the exam, or cancel the exam.
- If a decision is made to proceed, the physician will discuss with the patient the risk vs. benefits so that an informed decision can be made.
- All exams performed on pregnant patients will be documented on the requisition and in the report by the nuclear cardiologist.

Revised May 2001

---

## Example 4. Patient Identification Policy

Inpatients

- All inpatients must have a CCSS (hospital information system) request in their nuclear cardiology procedure folder.
- Check CCSS request to verify type of study you will be doing on the patient.
- Ask patient their first and last name, do not call them by name as a confused patient may answer yes incorrectly.
- Verify the patient's name by checking their ID bracelet. No exam should be performed on a patient without an ID bracelet.
- Have the fellow or nurse check the patient's hospital chart if any discrepancies arise.

Outpatients

- All outpatients should have a written request with them or have a faxed copy in their nuclear cardiology procedure folder.
- Verify patients first and last name.
- Ask the patient's birth date to verify the patient's identity.

If patients with similar names have procedures, take extra precaution for proper identification and attach colored notes to the chart to alert the physician who will be interpreting the study.
Revised December 2001

---

### *Example 5. Nuclear Cardiology Daily Survey Protocol*

- Area surveys must be performed each day that patients are imaged in the laboratory.
- On weekends and holidays, only surveys of the rooms actually used are necessary.
- All trash bins, linen hampers, and cold needle boxes must be surveyed in each imaging and stress room.
- Log the survey results in the Daily Room Survey Log book.
- Remember to record background activity and to check the battery of the survey meter.
- If any trash, linen, or needle boxes are found to be hot (twice back ground), they must be stored in the lead cabinet in the hot lab for decay. The box or bag is to be labeled with the date of storage.
- Any surface found to be contaminated or hot (twice background) must be cleaned and resurveyed. All cleaning should be done using gloves and blue absorbent pads to prevent further contamination. Collect all absorbent pads and gloves in trash bags to be held for decay in the lead cabinet in the hotlab. If the area still measures greater than 2 mR/h at 1 in., the area must be closed until sufficient decay occurs to bring the area into specifications. See Radioactive Spill Procedure or contact the RSO at 8-2950 for more details.
- Hot trash or contaminated areas should be brought to the attention of the chief technologist.
- The technologist performing the surveys must initial the logbook.

Revised October 2002

---

### *Example 6. Nuclear Cardiology Weekly Wipe Test Procedure*

| Tube # | Room # | Survey Area |
|--------|--------|-------------|
| 1 | | Background |
| 2 | | Background |
| 3 | | Background |
| 4 | Imaging room 1 | Imaging room 1 Floor |
| 5 | Imaging room 1 | Imaging room 1 Work Area |
| 6 | Imaging room 2 | Imaging room 2 Floor |

| 7  | Imaging room 2 | Imaging room 2 Work Area |
| 8  | Prep room 3    | Prep room Floor |
| 9  | Prep room 3    | Prep room Work Area |
| 10 | Imaging room 4 | Imaging room 4 Floor |
| 11 | Imaging room 4 | Imaging room 4 Work Area |
| 12 | Imaging room 5 | Imaging room 5 Floor |
| 13 | Imaging room 5 | Imaging room 5 Work Area |
| 14 | Imaging room 6 | Imaging room 6 Floor |
| 15 | Imaging room 6 | Imaging room 6 Work Area |
| 16 | Radiopharmacy  | Radiopharmacy Floor |
| 17 | Radiopharmacy  | Radiopharmacy Work Area (shield) |
| 18 | Radiopharmacy  | Radiopharmacy Work Area (sink) |
| 19 | Stress lab 1   | Stress lab 1 Floor |
| 20 | Stress lab 1   | Stress lab 1 Treadmill |
| 21 | Stress lab 2   | Stress lab 2 Left Floor |
| 22 | Stress lab 2   | Stress lab 2 Left Treadmill |
| 23 | Emergency      | Chest Pain Center Floor |
| 24 | Emergency      | Chest Pain Center Work Area |
| 25 | Emergency      | Chest Pain Center Treadmill |
| 26 |                | Cs-137 Test Source |
| 27 |                | Co-57 Test Source |

Wipe tests of all of the above areas must be done weekly. The assigned technologist is responsible for doing the weekly Wipes.

- Wipe the specified areas with Q-tips and insert them into the test tubes. Make sure the tube holder has the Protocol #20 clip on it and take to the Research lab to be counted in the well counter.
- Place the holder on the conveyer belt of the counter and hit F5 key to begin counting. The Protocol #20 clip will initiate the counter to run the wipe test protocol automatically.
- When the counting is complete, take the printout and check for contamination.
- Any areas found to be contaminated are to be cleaned following the steps in the radiation spill policy and re-wipe tested. If the wipe test is found to be clear, place it in the Weekly Wipe Test Manual located in the hotlab. If the area is still contaminated, the area must be closed off and re-tested in the morning prior to use.

Revised October 2002

# 19 Emergency Department Chest-Pain Center Imaging

In recent years many hospitals have instituted Chest Pain Centers (CPC) in hospital emergency departments (ED) for the purpose of efficient triage of patients with chest pain and normal or nonischemic rest ECG. The American Society of Nuclear Cardiology published a position paper on the use of radionuclide imaging in the ED (1) (on line www.asnc.org).

## PROTOCOL

The evaluation of patient with chest pain in a CPC typically involves two parts:

1. Rule out acute coronary syndrome (ACS) by acute rest SPECT imaging or serial assessment of biomarker for myocardial injury (CK, CK-MB, and troponin-I).
2. If ACS has been excluded, stress testing with or without SPECT imaging.
   Acute resting Tc-99m Sestamibi or Tc-99m-tetrofosmin imaging has high (99%) negative predictive value to exclude acute coronary syndrome (1,2). In a randomized controlled trial, resting Tc-99m Sestamibi perfusion imaging improved ED triage decision making and reduced unnecessary hospitalizations (3).

## LOCATION OF IMAGING

Although it is convenient, and perhaps preferable, to have a dedicated satellite stress/imaging laboratory on the ED premises, this is not a necessity. By design, patients evaluated in a CPC are low-risk patients. Higher-risk patients should be hospitalized. Thus, there is no serious patient safety concern with regard to transporting patients from the ED to a remote nuclear medicine laboratory in the hospital.

From: *Contemporary Cardiology: Nuclear Cardiology, The Basics*
F. J. Th. Wackers, W. Bruni, and B. L. Zaret © Humana Press Inc., Totowa, NJ

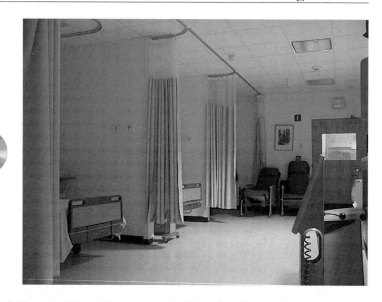

**Fig. 19-1.** Four-bed Chest Pain Center in Yale–New Haven Hospital.

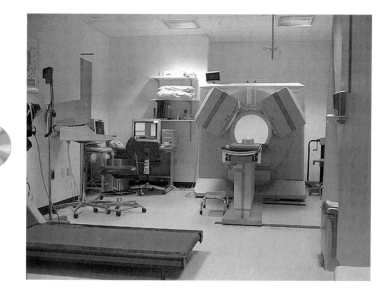

**Fig. 19-2.** Imaging and procedure room in the Yale–New Haven Hospital Chest Pain Center.

The most important difference between imaging in a CPC compared to imaging in the regular laboratory is that ED patients are unscheduled and present themselves 24 h a day, 7 d a week. This brings different logistic challenges into play.

## CHALLENGES FACED IN CHEST PAIN CENTERS

The following are challenges faced in chest pain centers:

- Staffing
    On-call 24/7
- Radiation safety
    Storage
    Injection, spill
- Patient safety
    Selection
    Emergencies
- Imaging protocol
    Acute rest imaging
    Optional stress imaging
- Timely interpretation
    Attending-on-call
    Communication with ED

### *Staffing*

A nuclear cardiologist and technologist should be on call during off-hours and weekends. For rest imaging the injection of radiopharmaceutical is preferably performed while the patient is still having pain, or < 2 h after pain has abated. Although some centers have arrangements for acute resting injection at any time, many centers have reached compromises with the ED and agreed on black out periods during the late evening and night when no imaging is performed.

Patients in whom an ACS has been excluded are eligible for stress testing. We found that "batch processing" of patients who are ready for stress testing works well for both patients and staff. In our CPC we perform stress tests with or without imaging in three periods:

- morning (around 9:00 AM)
- late afternoon (around 5:00 PM)
- evening (around 9:00 PM)

## *Radiation Safety*

In order to perform acute rest imaging 24 h per day in the ED, two options can be considered:

1. Preparation and radiolabeling of radiopharmaceutical kit in the ED facility. A dose can be drawn up when needed.
2. Ready-to-use unit doses delivered by commercial radiopharmacy.

Furthermore, the area used for radiotracer storage should have:

- Lead brick shielding and lead shield with glass for safe handling of radioactive material (**Fig. 19-3**).
- Dose calibrator for assaying and adjusting dose prior to injection.

Because the nuclear cardiology technologists on call generally are not on site during the off hours, it is useful if selected ED medical staff ("injectors") have received appropriate radiation safety training for injection of radiopharmaceuticals in patients with acute chest pain. This will enable patients to be injected during pain, instead of waiting for a technologist to arrive. When the technologist arrives, the patient will be ready to be imaged.

Radioactive spills are always a concern in a nuclear imaging facility. However, if the "injectors" are appropriately trained by the RSO, spills should not occur more frequently. The "injector" should have been trained in how to handle radioisotopes, and how to contain and decontaminate spills in the event one occurs.

## *Imaging Protocol*

### ACUTE REST IMAGING PROTOCOL

| | |
|---|---|
| Dose | 15 mCi, weight < 200 lb (< 90 kg) |
| | 25 mCi, weight > 200 lb (> 90 kg) |
| Time interval after injection | 30–45 min |
| Patient position | Supine |
| Imaging | Standard protocol (ECG gated) |
| Prone imaging | If inferior attenuation suspected |

### DISPOSITION AFTER ACUTE REST IMAGING IN CPC

| | |
|---|---|
| Normal: | Discharge home |
| | Optional stress testing |
| Abnormal: | Hospitalization |

Although studies have clearly shown that patients with normal acute rest SPECT images have an excellent short-term outcome, and thus can

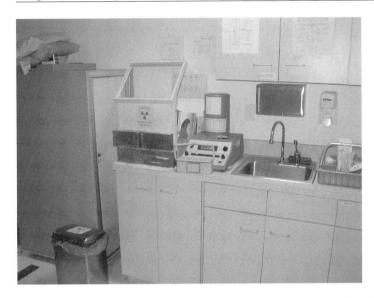

**Fig. 19-3.** Hot lab area in Chest Pain Center. The lead-shielded working area, dose calibrator fit on the counter top next to the zinc. Note wastebasket for radioactive waste.

be discharged when images are normal, some centers nevertheless perform stress testing prior to discharge.

Even when rest imaging or biomarkers of myocardial injury exclude acute coronary syndrome, patients may nevertheless have significant underlying coronary artery disease. A stress test prior to discharge is therefore useful to complete the cardiology work-up of patients with acute chest pain.

Radionuclide imaging plays an important role in this setting as approximately one-third of CPC patients cannot be evaluated by exercise ECG, because of inability to exercise, baseline ECG abnormalities that may preclude interpretation of ECG during exercise, or high pretest likelihood of coronary artery disease (4).

## *Stress Testing*

| | |
|---|---|
| Stress protocol | Standard Bruce Exercise ECG |
| | Standard Bruce Exercise Tc-99m- agent SPECT |
| | Adenosine vasodilation Tc-99m-agent SPECT |
| Dose | 25 mCi [if second dose after first low (15 mCi) dose, or next day in obese patients who had first high (25 mCi) dose] |

**Disposition after stress testing in a CPC:**

| | |
|---|---|
| Normal: | • Discharge home |
| Abnormal : | • Hospitalization, |
| | If only mildly abnormal consider: |
| | • Discharge home with arrangements for follow-up as out-patient |

## *Timely Interpretation*

Since the CPC is a 24/7 operation, rest imaging results and the results of stress tests must be communicated as soon as possible to the attending ED physicians. The nuclear cardiology attending serves as a consultant to the ED attending. Tele-nuclear cardiology (see Chapter 16) allows for remote reading of ECGs and nuclear images and is essential for the efficient operation of a CPC.

## SELECTED BIBILIOGRAPHY

1. Wackers FJTh, Brown KA, Heller GV, et al. (2002). American Society of Nuclear Cardiology position statement on radionuclide imaging in patients with suspected acute ischemic syndromes in the emergency department or chest pain center. *J Nucl Cardiol* 9:246–250.
2. Heller GV, Stowers SA, Hendel RC, et al. (1998). Clinical value of acute rest technetium-99m-tetrofosmin tomographic myocardial perfusion imaging in patients with acute chest pain and nondiagnostic electrocardiograms. *J Am Coll Cardiol* 31:1011–1017.
3. Udelson JE, Behansky JR, Ballin DS, et al. (2002). Myocardial perfusion imaging for evaluation and triage of patients with suspected acute cardiac ischemia. *JAMA* 288:2693–2700.
4. Abbott BG, Abdel-Aziz I, Nagula S, Monico EP, Schriver JA, Wackers FJTh (2001). Selective use of SPECT myocardial perfusion imaging in a chest pain center. *Am J Cardiol* 87:1351–1355.

# 20 Coding and Billing

Accurate coding and billing of procedures performed in the laboratory are extremely important. The following serves as a brief introduction to appropriate coding. However it is not the intention, nor is it possible, to provide definitive guidelines for any specific laboratory. Rules differ in different states and for different health maintenance providers. Always seek advice and check with local billing experts for accuracy.

## RECOMMENDED STEPS FOR APPROPRIATE CODING AND BILLING

- Credentialing Process
  1. Providers

     Providers must have current medical licenses, up-to-date curriculum vitae, records of CME credit hours, specialty board certifications (CBNC, ABR, and ABNM), diplomas, malpractice insurance, and, if a foreign medical school graduate, an Educational Commission for Foreign Medical School Graduate (ECFMG) certificate.

     To be eligible for reimbursement, more and more payers are now requiring CBNC-certification for nuclear cardiologists, as well as ICANL accreditation for laboratories.
  2. Payer participation

     If not familiar with contracts, employ someone who can contact insurers to find out if there are special requirements for billing for nuclear cardiology procedures. One should look to negotiate reimbursements and clearly understand the restrictions. A payer can have several plans and all will have separate rules. Create an index or guide for each payer to help alleviate questions at the time of patient appointment booking.
- Patient eligibility
  1. Referrals

     Verification that the patient belongs to a participating health maintenance organization.
  2. Payer authorizations

From: *Contemporary Cardiology: Nuclear Cardiology, The Basics*
F. J. Th. Wackers, W. Bruni, and B. L. Zaret © Humana Press Inc., Totowa, NJ

- Some payers require *pre-approval* of a test. For Medicare patients, no pre-approval is needed.
- Patient visit
  - Documentation
  - The nuclear cardiology report serves as documentation for visit
- Billing requirements
  1. Valid ICD-9 code(s)
  2. Appropriate CPT code(s)
  3. Appropriate modifiers
  4. Timely reporting
  5. Timely filing

---

**Fraud Awareness**

Providers must recognize their responsibility in complying with Medicare regulations. Medicare compliance requires that providers determine whether services they are furnishing are covered under the Medicare program. If services are not covered, providers should not submit a bill to Medicare.

---

## GENERAL PRINCIPLES

In order to receive reimbursement for diagnostic procedures, hard copy reports serve as documentation of services provided. Therefore, reports should contain all details necessary for appropriate coding. They should include the patient's diagnosis, indication for procedure (ICD-9 codes), and type(s) of procedure(s) performed (CPT codes). The procedural codes have a technical component and a professional component. It is important to note that the diagnosis code determines whether one receives reimbursement; the procedure code(s) determine at what level one is reimbursed. The diagnosis code(s) must fit the procedure code(s).

A complete list of CPT codes can be found in CPT reference books, i.e., CPT®Professional, which can be ordered online: http:// www.ingenixonline.com or by calling 1-800-Ingenix (464-3649). CPT codes are updated regularly. One should always use the most recent codes. The codes shown below were valid in the years 2002–2003.

Reimbursement may occur under two distinctly different conditions:

1. The provider is the sole owner of all equipment, e.g., physicians' office: technical, procedural, and interpretative billing are bundled in one (global fee).

**Table 20-1**
**A Few Examples of Useful ICD-9 Codes in Nuclear Cardiology**

| ICD9 codes | Item |
|---|---|
| 413.9 | Angina pectoris, other and unspecified |
| 786.50 | Chest pain unspecified |
| 414.8 | Other specific forms of chronic ischemic heart disease |
| 414.01 | Coronary atherosclerosis native coronary artery |
| 414.04 | Coronary atherosclerosis of artery bypass graft |
| 426.3 | Other left bundle branch block |
| 412 | Old myocardial infarction |
| 794.31 | Abnormal ECG |
| 411.89 | Other acute/subacute ischemic heart disease, Coronary insufficiency (acute), subendocardial ischemia |

2. The provider of services is *not* the owner of the equipment , e.g., within hospital setting: technical billing is separate from procedural and inter-pretative billing.

ICD9 codes are used to justify the performance of a particular procedure. A complete list of ICD-9 codes can be found in the ICD-9-CM reference book, i.e., ICD-9-CM for Physicians; volumes 1 & 2, which can be ordered online at: http://www.ingenixonline.com.

ICD9 codes are updated regularly. One should always use the most recent codes. The following codes were valid in 2002–2003.

Tables 20-1 and 20-2 list examples of ICD-9 and CPT codes.

Tables 20-3–20-7 show examples of appropriate coding for technical, professional, and supply components for ungated thallium stress SPECT imaging and for ECG-gated stress Tc-99m Sestamibi SPECT imaging. Note: For appropriate reimbursement the physician's report *must* state why pharmacological stress was used instead of treadmill exercise.

## CODING COMPLIANCE

It is important to create an internal coding compliance program that monitors appropriateness of coding and billing of the stress testing and imaging facility. When errors and possible violations are detected, they should be documented and appropriate course of action should be taken to avoid repetition.

**Table 20-2**
**CPT Codes for Nuclear Cardiology Procedures**

| CPT codes | Item |
|---|---|
| 78464 | Myocardial perfusion imaging SPECT: single study (i.e., stress or rest) |
| 78465 | Myocardial perfusion imaging SPECT: multiple studies (i.e., stress-rest, same day or two days) |
| 78478 add-on code, must be used with either 78464 or 78465 | Myocardial perfusion imaging (SPECT) with wall motion analysis |
| 78480 add-on code, must be used with either 78464 or 78465 | Myocardial perfusion imaging (SPECT) with ejection fraction assessment |
| 93016 | Cardiovascular stress test (MD supervision) |
| 93017 (not global) | Cardiovascular stress test (for obtaining ECG tracing only) |
| 93018 (not global) | Cardiovascular stress test ( for interpretation only) |
| 93015 (global) | Cardiovascular stress test ( global) |
| 78481 | First pass angiocardiography: single study |
| 78483 | First pass angiocardiography : multiple studies |
| 78472 | Cardiac blood pool imaging : single study |
| 78473 | Cardiac blood pool imaging : multiple studies |
| 78496 add-on code, must be used with 78472 | Cardiac blood pool imaging : single study with RVEF |
| 78494 | Cardiac blood pool imaging : single study SPECT |

*Warning*: the following codes should NEVER be used in combination, e.g., for dual isotope imaging (because it is fraud to bill twice):
　　78465 (SPECT MPI multiple studies) and:
　　78460   (Thallium MPI single study) or
　　78461   (Thallium MPI multiple studies) or
　　78464   (SPECT MPI single study)

Communication between physicians and billing staff is essential. There should be a voluntary compliance program with checks and balances. The physicians are responsible to ensure that provided services are reasonable and necessary. The coding and billing should match services provided and there should be proper documentation (i.e., request

**Table 20-3**
**Thallium-201 Stress SPECT Imaging**

| CPT codes | Item |
|---|---|
| *Technical component* | |
| 78465-TC | Myocardial perfusion imaging SPECT: multiple studies |
| 93015 (global, noTC) | Cardiovascular stress test |
| A9505 | Supply Tl-201: per mCi |
| *Professional component* | |
| 78465-26 | Myocardial perfusion imaging SPECT: multiple studies |
| 93016 | Cardiovascular stress test: MD supervision |
| 93018 | Cardiovascular stress test: interpretation/report NP: Nurse practioner code PA: Physician assistant code |

**Table 20-4**
**ECG-Gated Stress Sestamibi SPECT Imaging**

| CPT codes | Item |
|---|---|
| *Technical component* | |
| 78465-TC | Myocardial perfusion imaging SPECT scan: multiple studies |
| 93015 | Cardiovascular stress test |
| 78478-TC | Myocardial perfusion with wall motion |
| 78480-TC | Myocardial perfusion with ejection fraction |
| A9500 | Supply Tc99m Sestamibi:/dose |
| *Professional component* | |
| 78465-26 | Myocardial perfusion imaging SPECT: multiple studies |
| 93016 | CV stress test: MD supervision |
| 93018 | CV stress test: interpretation/report |
| 78478-26 | Myocardial perfusion with wall motion |
| 78465-26 | Myocardial perfusion with ejection fraction |

**Table 20-5**
**ECG-Gated Equilibrium Radionuclide Angiocardiography**

| CPT codes tech component | Item | CPT codes professional component | Item |
|---|---|---|---|
| 78472-TC | Gated blood pool imaging single study at rest | 78472 | Gated blood pool imaging single study at rest |
| 78473-TC | Gated blood pool imaging multiple studies (rest and stress) | 78473-26 | Gated blood pool imaging multiple studies (rest and stress) |
| A4641 | Supply of Tc-99m including Pyrophosphate or Ultratag® | | Red blood cell labeling (in vivo) Red blood cell labeling (in vitro) |

**Table 20-6**
**Codes for Supply of Radiopharmaceuticals**

| CPT codes | Item |
|---|---|
| A9505 | Thallium-201: per mCi |
| A9500 | Tc-99m-sestamibi: per dose |
| A9502 | Tc-99m-tetrofosmin: per dose |
| A4641 | Supply of radiopharmaceutical diagnostic imaging agent, not otherwise specified |
| 78990 | If provider does not accept "A" codes: provision of pharmaceutical |

**Table 20-7**
**Codes for Supply of Pharmaceuticals**

| HCPCS codes | Item |
|---|---|
| J1245 | Dipyridamole: per 10 mg |
| J0151 | Adenosine: per 90 mg unit (Adenoscan®) |
| J0150 | Adenosine: per 6 mg unit (Adenocard®) |
| J0280 | Aminophylline: up to 250 mg |
| J1250 | Dobutamine: per 250 mg |
| 99070 | If provider does not accept "J" codes: provision of pharmaceutical |

for services and detailed reports about services and results). Inappropriate coding and billing may result in decreased reimbursement and loss of revenues, and in addition, exposes the facility to the risk of audits.

We suggest that billing and compliance personnel acquire and reference the *National Correct Coding Primer with CorrectCodeChek*, published by Part B News Group. This useful reference book may serve as a guide for how to avoid denials for bundled codes and how to select correct coding combinations. One can obtain a copy of this manual that is updated quarterly by calling customer service at 1-877-397-1496, or on line at http://www.partbnews.com/pbnweb/resources.htm.

## QUESTIONS ABOUT REIMBURSEMENT

For Medicare reimbursement the local carriers should be able to answer most questions. In the case of third party payers, one may consult professionals at the payers' local or regional office. One can also call the ASNC Health Policy Director at (301) 493-2366 or email at boxall@asnc.org.

# 21 Laboratory Accreditation

Continuing quality assurance is an integral part of the present-day practice of medicine. Compliance by health care providers to quality standards set by organizations such as the Joint Commission on the Accreditation of Healthcare Organizations (JCAHO) is a matter of public record that can be carefully examined by the public as well as Health Maintenance Organizations (HMOs) and other health insurance providers. Throughout this book references have been made to standards of quality set by the Intersocietal Commission for Accreditation of Nuclear Laboratories (ICANL).

---

The ICANL was created in 1997 by experts in the field of nuclear cardiology to provide a mechanism for voluntary peer review of nuclear cardiology imaging facilities *(1)*.

At the time of this writing several HMOs have announced that ICANL accreditation will become mandatory in the near future for reimbursement for nuclear cardiology services (see also www.icanl.org).

## PURPOSE OF ACCREDITATION

The purpose of accreditation is twofold:

1. To set and provide realistic and well-defined objective standards of quality for nuclear laboratories.
2. To educate and assist laboratories in achieving this goal.

## TIME COMMITMENT

For a well-organized and well-run laboratory, it should not be difficult to obtain ICANL accreditation. This book contains a good deal of information about the material that is requested in an accreditation application. Well-written and detailed procedure protocols, evidence of

From: *Contemporary Cardiology: Nuclear Cardiology, The Basics*
F. J. Th. Wackers, W. Bruni, and B. L. Zaret © Humana Press Inc., Totowa, NJ

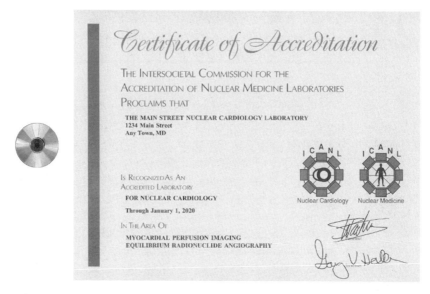

**Fig. 21-1.** Certificate of Accreditation in Nuclear Cardiology issued by the Intersocietal Commission for Accreditation of Nuclear Laboratories (ICANL)

QC and QA, good quality images, and clear reports are key elements that characterize a successful application for ICANL accreditation *(2)*. However, one should be willing to make the time commitment to put all the material together for a complete application. On an average, this work may take between 3–5 mo.

## COMPONENTS OF THE ICANL ACCREDITATION APPLICATION

The *Essentials and Standards* form the basis of the accreditation program. This comprehensive document provides standards for all aspects of patient testing and care, and was created following the classical triad of quality assessment: *Structure, Process, and Outcome*.

### Part I, Structure of Imaging Facility

In this part of the application the education, training, and credentials of the medical, technical, and other staff members are evaluated. In addition, the physical facilities, workload, equipment, and instrumentation must be described and listed. In order to be eligible for accreditation, an imaging facility should have been in existence for at least 1 yr and perform at least 300 studies per year.

## Part II, Process of Nuclear Cardiology

In this part of the application the degree of standardization of procedures is evaluated. Written protocols for all imaging and non-imaging procedures performed in the laboratory must be in place.

## Part III, Outcome and Quality Assurance

In this part of the application the quality of nuclear cardiology services and procedures are examined. This includes quality assurance of imaging and non-imaging equipment, quality assurance of imaging procedures and imaging results. The most important evaluation for accreditation involves peer review of randomly selected patient studies and the generated reports.

## REVIEW PROCESS

Two trained reviewers independently review each application. The reviewers objectively evaluate whether the submitted written material is in substantial compliance with the *Essentials and Standards*. An important component involves judging the quality of images and final reports. The reviewers each make an independent decision on the basis of the submitted material. The ICANL also conducts a site visit of every facility that applies for accreditation. These site visits primarily concentrate on the review of the camera and equipment quality control as well as all aspects of radiation safety. Both the application reviewers and the site visitor provide a report of significant findings and a recommendation to the ICANL Board of Directors, who review the submitted information and decide on the accreditation status of the laboratory.

Laboratories found to be in substantial compliance with the *Essentials and Standards* are granted accreditation for a 3-yr period. Laboratories that do not demonstrate substantial compliance with the *Essentials and Standards* receive the following decision(s): accreditation delayed pending correction of identified deficiencies and/or submissions of additional documents or accreditation denied. Any laboratory denied accreditation has the right to appeal the decision of the ICANL and may be re-evaluated by a new review panel.

## SELECTED BIBLIOGRAPHY

1. Wackers FJTh (1999). Blueprint of the Accreditation Program of the Intersocietal Commission for the Accreditation of Nuclear Medicine Laboratories. *J Nucl Cardiol* 6:372–374.
2. Wackers FJTh (2003). Accreditation of nuclear cardiology laboratories: an educational process. *J Nucl Cardiol* 10:205–207.

# INDEX

# ABOUT THE AUTHORS

Frans J. Th. Wackers is Professor of Diagnostic Radiology and Medicine and Director of the Cardiovascular Nuclear Imaging and Exercise Laboratories, Yale University School of Medicine, New Haven, CT.

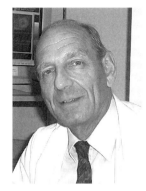

Born in Echt, The Netherlands, Dr. Wackers received both his MD and PhD degrees from the University of Amsterdam School of Medicine in 1970. He completed training in Internal Medicine and Cardiology in the former Wilhelmina Gasthuis, Amsterdam in 1977.

Dr. Wackers moved to the United States in 1977, where he was on the faculty of the Section of Cardiovascular Medicine at Yale University School of Medicine (1977–1981), the University of Vermont College of Medicine (1981–1984) and, since 1984, at Yale University School of Medicine.

Dr. Wackers is a Fellow of the American College of Cardiology; a Fellow of the American Heart Association, Council on Clinical Cardiology; a member of the Society of Nuclear Medicine; and a member of the American Society of Nuclear Cardiology. He is also a Diploma European Cardiologist of the European Society of Cardiology.

He is on the Editorial Board of the *Journal of the American College of Cardiology*, the *American Journal of Cardiology*, and *Journal of Nuclear Cardiology*. He was President of the Cardiovascular Council of The Society of Nuclear Medicine (1992–1993), President of the American Society of Nuclear Cardiology (1994–1995), President of the Certification Council of Nuclear Cardiology (1996–1997), and is currently President of the Intersocietal Commission for Accreditation of Nuclear Laboratories (1997–present).

Dr. Wackers is the recipient of the Rescar Award of the University of Maastricht, The Netherlands (1988); the Herrman Blumgart Award of the Society of Nuclear Medicine, New England Chapter (1995); the Homi Baba Award of the Indian Nuclear Cardiological Society (1997); the Eugene Drake Award of the American Heart Association, New England Affiliate (1999); and the Distinguished Service Award of the Society of Nuclear Cardiology (1999).

Dr. Wackers is considered a pioneer in Nuclear Cardiology. He is the founder of the American Society of Nuclear Cardiology (1993), the Certification Council of Nuclear Cardiology (1996), and the Intersocietal Commission for Accreditation of Nuclear Laboratories (1997). In 2003 he co-chaired the 6th International Conference of Nuclear Cardiology. He has published more than 270 articles on nuclear cardiology and clinical cardiology

Dr. Wackers is the Principal Investigator and Chairman of the multicenter ($n$=14) Detection of Ischemia in Asymptomatic Diabetics (DIAD) study. The study started in September 2000 and will continue until September 2007.

# ABOUT THE AUTHORS *(cont'd.)*

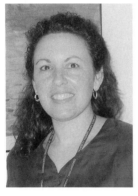

Wendy Bruni is chief technologist of Cardiovascular Nuclear Imaging Laboratory at Yale–New Haven Hospital, New Haven, CT. Ms. Bruni received a BS in nuclear medicine from the Rochester Institute of Technology, Rochester, NY in 1986. She worked in the nuclear medicine department at Community General Hospital, Syracuse, NY from 1986 to 1992. In 1992 she moved to Yale–New Haven Hospital, and since 1995 she has been the chief technologist of the nuclear cardiology department.

Ms. Bruni is an active member of the American Society of Nuclear Cardiology, participating on the technologist, newsletter, and program committees. She was secretary of the New England Chapter of the Society of Nuclear Medicine (1999) and chair of the Nuclear Cardiology Council of the Society of Nuclear Medicine Technologist Section. Ms. Bruni was selected to be on the panel of nuclear cardiology technologists who helped the NMTCB evaluate the Nuclear Cardiology Specialty Exam for technologists. She was one of the first to obtain the specialty certification of Nuclear Cardiology Technology (NCT) in June 2001.

Barry L. Zaret is Robert W. Berliner Professor of Medicine (Cardiovascular Medicine) and Professor of Diagnostic Radiology; Chief, Section of Cardiovascular Medicine; Associate Chair for Clinical Affairs, Department of Internal Medicine, Yale University School of Medicine, New Haven, CT.

Dr. Zaret received his BS degree from Queens College, City University of New York, and MD degree from New York University School of Medicine. He completed training in cardiology in 1971 at The Johns Hopkins University School of Medicine. Dr. Zaret became Chief of Cardiology at Yale University School of Medicine in 1978.

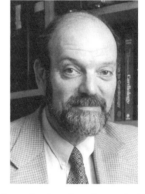

He is a Fellow of the American College of Cardiology, a Fellow of the American Heart Association, and a founding member of the American Society of Nuclear Cardiology. He is founding Editor-in-Chief of the *Journal of Nuclear Cardiology* and is on the Editorial Board of *Circulation,* the *Journal of the American College of Cardiology,* the *American Journal of Cardiology,* and the *Journal of Nuclear Cardiology.* He is a past President of the Association of Professors of Cardiology (1992–1993).

He has received a number of awards and recognitions, including: the Herrman Blumgart Award of the Society of Nuclear Medicine, New England Chapter (1978); the Louis Sudler Lecturer and Medalist, Rush-Presbyterian Medical College (1993); the Award for Contribution and Leadership in Noninvasive Cardiology, 4th International Conference on Noninvasive Cardiology, Cyprus (1993); the 29th Nathan J. Kiven Orator, Providence, RI (1996); The Solomon A. Berson Medical Alumni Achievement Award in Clinical Science, New York University School of Medicine (1998); Co-Chair 1st and 2nd International Conference of Nuclear Cardiology (1993, 1995), Co-Director, 2nd, 3rd, and 4th Wintergreen Conference on Nuclear Cardiology (1994, 1996, 1998); and First Samuel and Patsy Paine Lecturer, University of Texas (2001).

Dr. Zaret is considered one of the founders and present leaders of the subspecialty of nuclear cardiology. He has made numerous contributions to the cardiology literature on myocardial perfusion imaging and assessment of cardiac function using radionuclide imaging methodology.

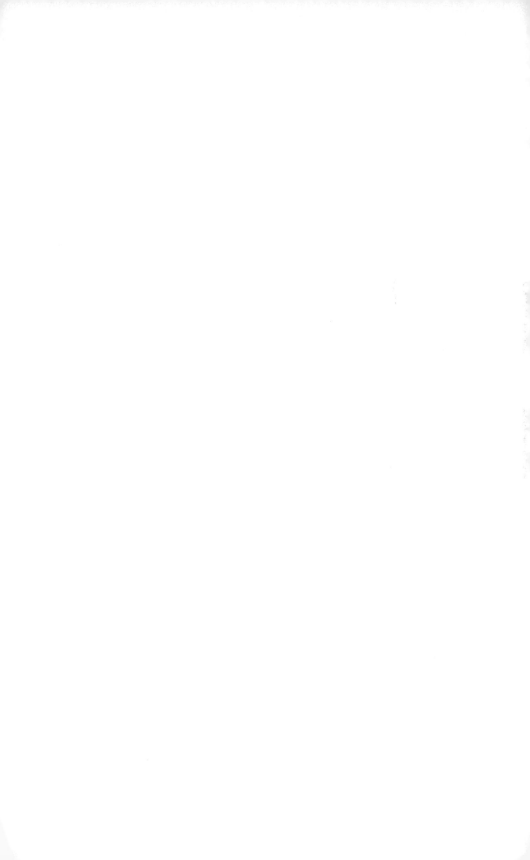